Psychological Treatment of
**Medical Patients
Struggling With
Harmful Substance Use**

Clinical Health Psychology Series

Psychological Treatment of
Medical Patients Struggling With Harmful Substance Use

JULIE A. SCHUMACHER and DANIEL C. WILLIAMS

CLINICAL HEALTH PSYCHOLOGY SERIES

ELLEN A. DORNELAS, Series Editor

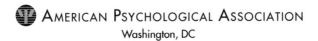 AMERICAN PSYCHOLOGICAL ASSOCIATION
Washington, DC

Published by
American Psychological Association
750 First Street, NE
Washington, DC 20002
https://www.apa.org

Order Department
https://www.apa.org/pubs/books
order@apa.org

In the U.K., Europe, Africa, and the Middle East, copies may be ordered from Eurospan
https://www.eurospanbookstore.com/apa
info@eurospangroup.com

Typeset in Charter and Interstate by Circle Graphics, Inc., Reisterstown, MD

Printer: Sheridan Books, Chelsea, MI
Cover Designer: Mercury Publishing Services, Inc., Rockville, MD

Library of Congress Cataloging-in-Publication Data
Names: Schumacher, Julie A., author.
Title: Psychological treatment of medical patients struggling with harmful substance use / Julie A. Schumacher & Daniel C. Williams.
Description: Washington : American Psychological Association, [2020] | Series: Clinical health psychology series | Includes bibliographical references and index.
Identifiers: LCCN 2019022627 (print) | LCCN 2019022628 (ebook) | ISBN 9781433830785 (paperback) | ISBN 9781433831683 (ebook)
Subjects: LCSH: Substance abuse—Psychological aspects. | Psychotherapy. | Physician and patient.
Classification: LCC RC564 .S335 2020 (print) | LCC RC564 (ebook) | DDC N 616.86/0651—dc23
LC record available at https://lccn.loc.gov/2019022627
LC ebook record available at https://lccn.loc.gov/2019022628

http://dx.doi.org/10.1037/0000160-000

Printed in the United States of America

10 9 8 7 6 5 4 3 2 1

Contents

Series Foreword

Mental health practitioners working in medicine represent the vanguard of psychological practice. As scientific discovery and advancement in medicine has rapidly evolved in recent decades, it has been a challenge for clinical health psychology practice to keep pace.

In a fast-changing field, and with a paucity of practice-based research, classroom models of health psychology practice often don't translate well to clinical care. All too often, health psychologists work in silos, with little appreciation of how advancement in one area might inform another. The goal of the Clinical Health Psychology series is to change these trends and provide a comprehensive yet concise overview of the essential elements of clinical practice in specific areas of health care. The future of 21st-century health psychology depends on the ability of new practitioners to be innovative and to generalize their knowledge across domains. To this end, the series focuses on a variety of topics and provides both a foundation as well as specific clinical examples for mental health professionals who are new to the field.

Working with Susan Reynolds, senior acquisitions editor at APA Books, I am very proud to have had an opportunity to edit this book series. We have chosen authors who are recognized experts in the field and are rethinking the practice of health psychology to be aligned with modern drivers of health care, such as population health, cost of care, quality of care, and the patient experience.

Psychological Treatment of Medical Patients Struggling With Harmful Substance Use by Julie A. Schumacher and Daniel C. Williams provides mental health practitioners with essential information about how to recognize substance use in people treated in medical settings. Behavioral health clinicians working in primary and specialty care settings often encounter patients who are prescribed stimulants, sedatives, and/or opioid analgesics to treat common problems such as sleep disturbance, pain, anxiety, and fatigue. Substance abuse is associated with stigma, and it can be difficult for both patients and their medical providers to conceptualize that many drugs with therapeutic benefit can also be a source of substance use disorder ranging on a continuum from mild to severe. The authors skillfully guide readers through an overview of a long neglected topic and provide clinical case examples to illustrate the material. Referral to specialty substance abuse clinics is often neither practical nor appropriate for patients with substance use disorders encountered in medical or private practice mental health settings. This concise and contemporary volume packs a wealth of evidence-based practical information on screening, assessment, and treatment of this patient population. We are pleased to include this book in APA's Clinical Health Psychology series. It is sure to become a frequently used resource for practicing clinical health psychologists.

—*Ellen A. Dornelas, PhD*
Series Editor

Psychological Treatment of
Medical Patients
Struggling With
Harmful Substance Use

INTRODUCTION

"Because of the prevalence of substance abuse in general clinical populations, it is important for psychologists to have knowledge and skill in this area" (p. 1269). This is the first line of the abstract for Miller and Brown's (1997) article, "Why Psychologists Should Treat Alcohol and Drug Problems," published in *American Psychologist*. Flash forward more than 20 years and many psychologists still receive little to no training in substance use disorders or other forms of harmful substance use. Findings of a longitudinal survey of directors of clinical training in American Psychological Association (APA)–accredited U.S. clinical psychology doctoral programs published in 2017 in *American Psychologist* found that "less than 40% of programs had even 1 faculty member studying addiction, and less than one third offered any specialty clinical training in addiction," and that number had not increased over the 14-year study period (Dimoff, Sayette, & Norcross, 2017, p. 689). There is evidence that a similar situation exists in counseling and counseling psychology programs (Madson, Bethea, Daniel, & Necaise, 2008; J. L. Martin, Burrow-Sánchez, Iwamoto, Glidden-Tracey, & Vaughan, 2016).

Clinical health psychologists and other mental health professionals working in a variety of medical settings from primary care to the emergency

http://dx.doi.org/10.1037/0000160-001
Psychological Treatment of Medical Patients Struggling With Harmful Substance Use, by J. A. Schumacher and D. C. Williams

department are very likely to encounter patients who would benefit from interventions for substance use. Even patients engaging in substance use who might otherwise be considered low risk may be placing themselves at risk; almost 42% of U.S. adults who drink also report taking medications known to interact with alcohol (Breslow, Dong, & White, 2015). In addition, a number of medical conditions increase risk for or complicate treatment of substance use problems or are caused or worsened by substance use. Moreover, one of the fastest growing areas of harmful substance use in the United States is nonmedical prescription drug use (Substance Abuse and Mental Health Services Administration, 2013), which may begin with a therapeutic prescription (Canfield et al., 2010). For these reasons, it is essential that clinical health psychologists and other mental health professionals working in medical settings have some comfort with assessing and addressing substance use issues.

The goal of this book is to equip such professionals with a basic level of knowledge and skills in the spectrum of substance use encountered in a variety of outpatient medical settings. Although written specifically with clinical health psychologists in mind, given the varied and overlapping roles of mental health professionals in medical settings, particularly in rural areas, this book is also relevant for other psychologists and mental health professionals in medical settings. The book provides information to help providers (a) speak more knowledgeably with their patients and other providers about various aspects of alcohol and drug use; (b) recognize variations in alcohol and drug use etiology and epidemiology in different clinical settings; and (c) adequately assess alcohol and drug use and make appropriate referrals when intervention is necessary. For providers who already have some background knowledge, this book provides ideas about how to incorporate interventions for alcohol and drug use into other treatment plans when specialty care is not necessary and to assess and treat three commonly co-occurring conditions: depression, anxiety, and sleep problems. More generally, this book seeks to bolster providers' awareness of and confidence in addressing alcohol and drug use in whatever setting they practice. This will increase the chances that patients who are engaging in harmful substance use do not fall through the cracks and instead receive the types of care they need.

Topics beyond the scope of the current book are harmful substance use in the context of pain management, harmful substance use in adolescents, sexual dysfunction, and co-occurring personality disorders and serious mental disorder. We also decided to exclude tobacco use even though it is included in the fifth edition of the *Diagnostic and Statistical Manual of Mental Disorders* (*DSM–5*) as a substance-related disorder.

Tobacco assessment and treatment are important and deserving of focused attention. For current recommendations for tobacco cessation for adults, see *Final Recommendation Statement: Tobacco Smoking Cessation in Adults, Including Pregnant Women: Behavioral and Pharmacotherapy Interventions* from the U.S. Preventive Services Task Force (2019; available at https://www.uspreventiveservicestaskforce.org/Page/Document/Recommendation StatementFinal/tobacco-use-in-adults-and-pregnant-women-counseling-and-interventions1).

OUR MOTIVATION FOR WRITING THIS BOOK

Our personal motivation for writing this book comes from our own professional journeys as psychologists working with individuals experiencing various harms related to alcohol and drugs. We've seen individuals with multiple nonfatal overdoses who find themselves in treatment once again trying to gain the knowledge and skills that will help them avoid falling back into the trap of addiction, perhaps while also trying to manage chronic pain. We've seen individuals who have experienced a driving under the influence arrest and are grappling with the substantial legal, financial, and social ramifications of this one event and hoping to prevent a recurrence. We've seen individuals who have been told by their physician that if they do not stop drinking, they will likely die from alcohol-related disease. We've seen individuals who smoke marijuana daily because they believe it is a completely safe drug with no risk for addiction or other ill effects. Through these and many other individuals with whom we've had the privilege to work, we've seen the alcohol and drug epidemiology come to life in real human beings. We have learned that in every clinical setting, if we ask the right questions and know what to look for, we will find individuals who are at risk for harms related to alcohol and drugs, individuals who are already experiencing harms related to alcohol and drugs, and individuals who are held tight within the grip of a severe substance use disorder. Most importantly, we know firsthand that psychologists in medical settings have tremendous potential to improve the lives of these individuals through direct care, appropriate referral, advocacy, and teaching.

OVERVIEW OF THE BOOK

Below we provide a brief overview of each of the chapters in this book for readers who are interested in using the book as a quick reference guide rather than reading it in its entirety. Readers who have limited experience with harmful substance use are encouraged to read the first three chapters before proceeding to subsequent chapters.

Part I: Overview of Substance Use

Part I provides a broad overview of substance use and substance use disorders that is specifically tailored for psychologists working with medical patients.

Chapter 1 is an easy-to-read reference guide that will give mental health professionals a basic working knowledge of the distinction between substance use and harmful substance use as well as the signs and symptoms of substance use disorders.

Chapter 2 includes an introduction to epidemiology and current models of the biological and sociocultural causes of and contributing factors to harmful substance use, with an emphasis on cardiac, cancer, women's health, and primary care settings, where clinical health psychologists are commonly involved in patient care.

Chapter 3 provides an overview of best-practice assessment strategies and typical psychological, self-help, and pharmacological treatment for harmful substance use, including information about the research support for these treatments and referral guidelines.

Chapter 4 concludes this first section with detailed information about implementing assessment and brief intervention for harmful substance use in medical settings, including practical guidance for implementing Screening Brief Intervention and Referral to Treatment (SBIRT), an evidence-based tool for addressing harmful substance use and addiction in nonspecialty settings.

Part II: Psychological Assessment and Intervention for Common Comorbid Problems

Part II of the book focuses on strategies for addressing psychological problems that commonly co-occur with harmful substance use, as well as strategies for addressing the needs of families and addressing the needs of patients who have completed specialty substance use disorder treatment. Each of the chapters ends with a clinical vignette to illustrate application of key concepts and strategies in a patient receiving treatment in a primary care, cancer, cardiac care, or women's health setting. The vignettes are fictional composites of typical patients.

Chapter 5 describes the complex, reciprocal relationships between depression and harmful substance use and provides practical guidance on assessing depression in patients with harmful substance and a summary of evidence-based psychotherapeutic approaches to treating patients with these co-occurring problems.

Chapter 6 provides recommendations for assessing anxiety and trauma-related disorders that co-occur with harmful substances, discusses mechanisms of co-occurrence among these disorders, and presents a continuum of evidence-based treatments for anxiety and related disorders for patients with harmful substance use.

Chapter 7 focuses on assessment and treatment of sleep dysregulation, which is common in patients with harmful substance use and can persist after substance use ceases, and offers information on how to assess and treat co-occurring sleep problems.

Chapter 8 turns attention to psychological treatment of family members who are dealing with a loved one's harmful substance use including information about the efficacy of widely available and lesser known approaches.

Part II concludes with a focus on relapse prevention and continuing care in Chapter 9 and presentation of common evidence-based behavioral relapse prevention approaches.

The book concludes with a more detailed description of why clinical health psychologists and other mental health professionals who work with medical patients need to become more adept at addressing harmful substance use, and it addresses aspects of care delivery that would promote better integration between the psychological and medical care of the medical patient with harmful substance use. Future directions for practice and training are also discussed.

PART I OVERVIEW OF SUBSTANCE USE

1 MENTAL HEALTH PROFESSIONALS' GUIDE TO UNDERSTANDING HARMFUL SUBSTANCE USE

Confusion is common about what constitutes harmful substance use and addiction. On the one hand, there are some reports that moderate amounts of alcohol can be beneficial. More and more states are legalizing marijuana for medical or recreational use. Heavy drinking is common on college campuses. On the other hand, the dangers of alcohol and drugs are readily apparent in society, through drug overdoses, drunk driving, and health problems. It's not surprising, then, that most laypeople are unsure of the guidelines surrounding low-risk drinking and drug use. Many providers are also unsure of what to recommend to patients with the literature and popular media filled with seemingly contradictory points of information.

This chapter is written with clinicians who are not experts in substance use assessment and treatment in mind. It is intended as an easy-to-read reference guide that will give mental health professionals a basic working knowledge of the distinction between substance use and harmful substance use as well as the signs and symptoms of substance use disorders.

http://dx.doi.org/10.1037/0000160-002
Psychological Treatment of Medical Patients Struggling With Harmful Substance Use,
by J. A. Schumacher and D. C. Williams

TERMINOLOGY

We begin with definitions of terms that are used in substance use treatment. Terms such as *alcoholic* and *addict* are commonly used in everyday language, but they are likely to feel judgmental to patients. The exception to this rule is that some patients, many of whom are actively involved in 12-step programs, have embraced these terms as part of their recovery. We recommend allowing patients to dictate the terms by which they are identified.

Other terms that are used in the literature are defined here for your reference:

- *Substance use disorder:* Meeting *Diagnostic and Statistical Manual of Mental Disorders, Fifth Edition* (*DSM–5*; American Psychiatric Association, 2013a) criteria for a substance-related disorder.

- *Substance abuse:* Old *DSM–IV* (American Psychiatric Association, 2000) terminology, now referred to as a *use disorder*.

- *Substance dependence:* Old *DSM–IV* terminology, now referred to as a use disorder. Currently used by the *International Statistical Classification of Diseases and Related Health Problems* (ICD–10; World Health Organization, 1992) for a use disorder.

- *Physiological dependence:* Alcohol, most illicit drugs, and some medications, even when taken as prescribed, can lead to tolerance and withdrawal.

- *Binge drinking:* Males consuming five or more drinks per occasion, females consuming four or more drinks per occasion.

- *Low-risk drinking:* Males consuming no more than four drinks per day, 14 drinks per week. Females consuming no more than three drinks per day, seven drinks per week.

- *At-risk substance use:* For alcohol, drinking more than the low-risk drinking guidelines. For drugs, any use of illicit drugs, taking medications not as prescribed.

- *Hazardous substance use:* A term used by the World Health Organization for use that increases the risk of negative consequences to the user, but sub-threshold for a substance use disorder.

- *Harmful substance use:* A term used by the ICD–10 for a pattern of use that is causing damage to health physically or mentally.

SUBSTANCE USE DISORDER DIAGNOSTIC CRITERIA

Many psychologists who have been in practice for some time are familiar with the distinction within *DSM–IV* between *substance abuse* and *substance dependence*. Previously, substance use disorders were thought to fall within two categories—abuse and dependence—with abuse being less severe and dependence being more severe. Research on substance use and the problems that develop as a result of chronic substance use, however, did not support this binary distinction (Hasin et al., 2013). Instead, research supports thinking of substance use disorders on a continuum—a conceptualization that was adopted for *DSM–5*. Within this framework, the severity level is determined on the basis of the number of diagnostic criteria met: Two to three criteria are classified as a mild disorder, while four to five is considered moderate, and six or more is classified as severe. Although the overarching conceptualization of substance use disorders transitioned from a categorical to a continuous framework, with two exceptions noted below, the symptom criteria are largely identical between *DSM–IV* and *DSM–5*.

According to *DSM–5*, the 11 criteria for diagnosing substance use disorders can be thought of as grouping within four broad categories: impaired control, social impairment, risky use, and pharmacological symptoms. Craving, long recognized as an associated feature of substance use disorders, is a new symptom criterion in the impaired control category introduced in *DSM–5*. Craving is a key reason that the continuing care and relapse prevention strategies discussed in Chapter 9, this volume, may be important for many patients following initial treatment for a substance use disorder; craving is a symptom that may persist well into periods of abstinence. Recurrent substance-related legal problems, which were a symptom criterion for *DSM–IV* substance abuse, are excluded from the *DSM–5* social impairment category. The criteria in the risky use and pharmacological symptoms categories were all maintained from *DSM–IV*.

As in *DSM–IV*, assigning the symptom criterion of withdrawal requires that either the individual meets the criteria for the withdrawal syndrome for that substance as specified in *DSM–5* or the individual takes a substance to relieve or avoid withdrawal. Withdrawal syndromes are specified for alcohol and all drugs except inhalants and hallucinogens. Knowledge of withdrawal symptoms is an important competency for psychologists and all mental health providers given the high prevalence of substance use disorder and the risk for serious and even life-threatening withdrawal symptoms associated with substances such as alcohol and benzodiazepines if withdrawal is not completed under appropriate medical supervision. When in doubt, refer to a medical colleague for evaluation of withdrawal symptoms (see Wood et al., 2018, for a medical review of alcohol withdrawal assessment).

In considering whether a patient meets criteria for a substance use disorder, it is important to note that tolerance and withdrawal are expected to occur with appropriate medical use of some prescription medications, such as benzodiazepines and opioid analgesics. When these symptoms occur within the context of appropriate medical treatment, they are not considered toward diagnosing a substance use disorder. For example, if a patient with panic disorder is prescribed a benzodiazepine and takes it consistently, it would be expected that over time the original dose would not have the same anxiolytic effect and the patient may require higher doses to maintain the original response. It would also be expected that if the patient abruptly stopped taking the medication, there would be physiological withdrawal symptoms, such as sweating, insomnia, anxiety, agitation, and even seizures (American Psychiatric Association, 2013a). However, in the absence of use of the benzodiazepine that was in excess of prescribed amounts or that resulted in other symptoms of substance use disorder, a substance use disorder would not be diagnosed.

Given that the *International Classification of Disorders* (ICD; World Health Organization, 1992) is used for billing purposes, it also is important for clinicians to be familiar with their classification system as well. The ICD is created by the World Health Organization in order to have a universal diagnostic classification system and classifies substance use disorders as "mental and behavioral disorders due to psychoactive substance use." ICD terminology is different than both *DSM–IV* and *DSM–5* classifications, instead using the term *harmful use* to refer to *DSM–IV abuse* and the term *dependence syndrome* to refer to *DSM–IV dependence*.

HAZARDOUS AND HARMFUL SUBSTANCE USE

The *DSM–5* does not have any criteria related to quantity of use or specify guidelines for low-risk alcohol or drug use. Nonetheless, many patients who do not meet diagnostic criteria for a substance use disorder may use drugs and alcohol in ways that place them at risk for acute accidents or injuries, chronic diseases, or developing substance use disorders. They also may use substances as a way of regulating their emotional responses to other psychiatric disorders or previous traumatic experiences. Thus, it is also important for clinicians to be able to identify and intervene with patients engaging in hazardous or harmful substance use who do not meet *DSM–5* diagnostic criteria.

Alcohol

Because there is general consensus that for most patients some amount of alcohol may be consumed without substantially increasing risk for alcohol-related problems, several factors must be considered in determining whether a particular patient's alcohol use is problematic. Next, we outline the factors and guidelines that must be considered in evaluating a particular patient's risk level.

Standard Drink Conversion

Different kinds of alcoholic drinks containing different amounts of alcohol can be consumed in a variety of different quantities. To have a standardized metric for comparison, a "standard drink" has been established (National Institute on Alcohol Abuse and Alcoholism [NIAAA], 2010). One standard drink is equivalent to 14 grams of ethanol, which is 12 ounces of beer (5% alcohol content), 5 ounces of wine (12% alcohol content), or 1.5 ounces of liquor (40% alcohol content or 80 proof). The drinking guidelines presented here use standard drinks as the basis for their recommendations (see Exhibit 1.1).

Low-Risk Drinking Guidelines

NIAAA (2010) has established low-risk drinking guidelines. These guidelines are adjusted for age and sex and focus on both daily and weekly limits for drinking. For men between ages 21 and 65, low-risk drinking is defined

---

EXHIBIT 1.1. Tips for Assessing Alcohol Consumption

When assessing for alcohol use, it is important to translate what a patient considers one drink to standard drinks to objectively determine whether the patient is drinking within recommended limits. If a patient reports drinking "three beers," but each beer is 22 ounces, then the patient is actually consuming nearly six standard drinks. Here are a few practical tips when working with patients:

- When asking about alcohol use, show a picture of standard drink conversions so that the patient can visually understand.
- Mixed drinks contain other beverages, such as soda or juice, in addition to alcohol. If you don't subtract the other beverages from the alcohol in your calculation, you will overestimate the amount of alcohol in the drink.
- "Solo" cups—the colored cups often used at parties—have lines designating standard drinks and can be a useful comparison for estimating alcohol with patients.

as no more than four standard drinks per day and no more than 14 standard drinks per week. For women, low-risk drinking is no more than three drinks per day and no more than seven drinks per week. For men 65 and older, low-risk drinking guidelines reduce in quantity to no more than three drinks per day and no more than seven drinks per week. Research shows that drinking at this level, only 2% of individuals will develop an alcohol use disorder (NIAAA, 2010).

To stay within low-risk drinking guidelines, both the daily and weekly limits must be kept. The daily limits are primarily focused on the dangers inherent in physical and cognitive impairment resulting from increasing blood alcohol levels and are designed to prevent drinkers from reaching blood alcohol concentration at the 0.08 level. Drinking at this level increases risk for injuries, such as car accidents, falls, burns, and drownings. It also increases risk for risky behaviors, such as unprotected sex, sexual assault, and violence. The weekly limits, on the other hand, are focused on the accumulative negative effects from drinking. These include a variety of health problems, such as liver and heart disease, sleep disorders, stroke, cancer, and the management of chronic conditions such as diabetes or hypertension. Chronic violation of the low-risk guidelines also increases risk for developing an alcohol use disorder.

Binge Drinking

Binge drinking, according to the NIAAA (2010), is defined as drinking that leads to a blood alcohol concentration of 0.08g/dL, which is generally the DUI limit in many states (NIAAA, 2010). The National Survey on Drug Use and Health defines binge drinking as four or more standard drinks for women, and five or more standard drinks for men, on the same occasion (Center for Behavioral Health Statistics and Quality, 2016). Binge drinking is associated with a variety of health complications and injuries (World Health Organization, 2014), such as car accidents, falls, burns, domestic violence, sexual assault, sexually transmitted diseases, fetal alcohol spectrum disorders, a variety of cancers, chronic health conditions such as diabetes and hypertension, cognitive problems, and alcohol use disorder.

People Who Should Not Drink at All

For individuals with some health conditions, abstinence from drinking is recommended. That includes individuals under age 21, pregnant women, and individuals with liver problems such as hepatitis C or cirrhosis. Individuals who plan to operate a vehicle or engage in activities that require full levels of coordination should abstain from alcohol. Also, a large number of medications—both prescribed and over the counter—interact with alcohol in dangerous ways. Common classes of medications, which interact with alcohol in problematic ways, include nonsteroidal anti-inflammatory drugs, antibiotics, anticonvulsants, antihistamines, anticoagulants, benzodiazepines, and antidiabetic agents (Weathermon & Crabb, 1999). For example, alcohol and acetaminophen interact to increase toxicity to the liver. Patients prescribed medications with negative alcohol interactions are commonly unaware of this potential problem (R. L. Brown, Dimond, Hulisz, Saunders, & Bobula, 2007).

Underage Drinking

Findings from the Youth Risk Behavior Surveillance System (Grunbaum et al., 2004) show that drinking under the age of 21 is common in the United States with 74.9% of students in Grades 9 through 12 having had one or more drinks of alcohol on at least one day in their lifetime and 44.9% within the past month. Having five or more drinks of alcohol within a short period of time occurred in the past month for 28.3% of ninth-graders through 12th-graders surveyed. Underage drinking is particularly risky for the developing brain (Crews, He, & Hodge, 2007) and is associated with a variety of negative consequences (Hingson & White, 2014), such as increased risk of dying in a car accident, substance overdoses, cognitive impairment, and substantial economic costs. Underage drinking that exceeds guidelines for adults greatly increases the odds of having clinically significant anxiety, depression, and suicidal ideation (Richter, Pugh, Peters, Vaughan, & Foster, 2016).

Moderate Drinking Guidelines

In addition to the NIAAA low-risk drinking guidelines, the U.S. Department of Health and Human Services and the U.S. Department of Agriculture (2015) have developed guidelines for moderate drinking. These guidelines are embedded within a broader set of dietary guidelines designed to prevent chronic health-related problems. Given the caloric content of alcohol and the health-related problems that excessive alcohol use can cause, moderate drinking guidelines have been developed in order to maintain a healthy lifestyle. One standard drink, based purely on alcohol, contains 98 calories. Most alcohol beverages contain more calories due to the addition of other ingredients. For example, a 12-oz beer has about 150 calories, 5 oz of wine has about 120 calories, and adding fruit juice or soda to liquor (e.g., rum and coke) adds additional calories. As a result, drinking can easily lead to unhealthy caloric intake if not monitored.

Based on these dietary factors, moderate drinking is defined as one standard drink per day for women and two standard drinks per day for men.

They also recommend that nondrinkers don't start drinking for any reason. They define high-risk drinking as any drinking higher than the daily or weekly limits outlined by NIAAA above.

Drugs

While drug use disorders occur much less frequently than alcohol use disorders, drug use is much more common than many realize. Nearly half of all individuals ages 12 and older, in the United States, have used illicit drugs or misused prescription medications in their lifetime (Center for Behavioral Health Statistics and Quality, 2016). The remainder of this chapter briefly reviews the use of illegal drugs and the misuse of over-the-counter drugs and prescription medications. Currently established guidelines encourage abstinence from all illicit drugs, including marijuana, or misuse of over-the-counter or prescription medications (National Institute on Drug Abuse, 2012b).

Illicit Drug Use

We use the term *illicit drugs* to refer to drugs that are illegal to use or possess according to U.S. law. At the writing of this book, that includes marijuana under most circumstances. Illicit drug use is highest among emerging adults (ages 18–25; Substance Abuse and Mental Health Services Administration, 2017).

Marijuana. The mostly commonly used illicit drug is marijuana. As reviewed in the recent landmark report of the National Academies of Science, Engineering, and Medicine (2017) titled *The Health Effects of Cannabis and Cannabinoids: The Current State of Evidence and Recommendations for Research*, marijuana is derived from the Cannabis sativa plant. This plant contains more than 100 chemical compounds called cannabinoids. The only compound in marijuana that makes people feel "high" is tetrahydrocannabinol (THC). The potency of cannabis has been increasing over the past 2 decades from approximately 4% THC in 1995 to 12% THC in 2014, and strains of cannabis with higher THC levels are increasingly available. The term *medical marijuana*, particularly when it appears in popular media, is somewhat confusing because it is often used to refer to marijuana, specific cannabinoids or cannabinoid combinations, and even synthetic cannabinoids. Most studies of the potential medical uses of marijuana or marijuana derivatives do not focus on smoked marijuana. Instead, much of this research focuses on one to two isolated cannabinoids or synthetic cannabinoids, which may or may not include THC (National Academies of Science, Engineering, & Medicine, 2017). Thus, it is important for psychologists and other health-care providers to read this research carefully, so they are equipped to address the many questions patients may have or comments they may make about "medical marijuana."

Attitudes toward marijuana use have evolved over time, with many states loosening regulations for medical or recreational use of marijuana. None-theless, there are a variety of risks associated with marijuana use (National Academies of Science, Engineering, & Medicine, 2017; Volkow, Baler, Compton, & Weiss, 2014). Short-term negative effects include impaired short-term memory, impaired motor coordination, increased risk of acute myo-cardial infarction, altered judgment, and paranoia and psychosis in high doses. Long-term consequences include altered brain development, increased likelihood of dropping out of school, cognitive impairment, diminished life satisfaction and achievement, symptoms of chronic bronchitis, and increased risk of a chronic psychotic disorder in individuals predisposed to psychosis. There is also evidence that regular or heavy marijuana use may increase symptoms of mania and hypomania in individuals with bipolar disorders and increase suicide attempt and completion. Despite its reputation as a "safe drug," the risk of addiction exists as well, with about 10% of indi-viduals who experiment with cannabis becoming daily users, and 20% to 30% becoming weekly users (Hall & Degenhardt, 2009). While the risk for developing a cannabis use disorder is lower than other drugs, it is still significant. Research shows that about 9% of cannabis users in the United States will eventually develop a cannabis use disorder (Anthony, 2006; Anthony, Warner, & Kessler, 1994). Rates increase to 16% for those who initiate use as an adolescent (Anthony, 2006), and a 3-year prospective study of daily cannabis users 18 and older revealed that 37% developed dependence (van der Pol et al., 2013). This stands in stark contrast to public perceptions of the safety of cannabis use, where only 34% of people age 12 and older perceive weekly use of marijuana to be a "great risk" (Lipari, Ahrnsbrak, Pemberton, & Porter, 2017).

Hallucinogens. Hallucinogens are substances that create significant distor-tions in a person's perceptions of reality (National Institute on Drug Abuse, 2015). This class includes classic hallucinogens, such as d-lysergic acid diethylamide (LSD) and mescaline (peyote), as well as dissociative drugs such as phencyclidine (PCP), salvia, and ketamine. Some hallucinogens do not have an established withdrawal syndrome, but tolerance is often quickly developed. Although some of the short-term effects of hallucinogens are described as pleasurable, aversive psychological and physiological reactions may occur, including panic and fear, anxiety, paranoia, and aggression. Negative long-term effects include ongoing psychotic symptoms (e.g., disorganized thinking, paranoia), as well as hallucinogen persisting perception disorder (i.e., ongoing reexperiencing of hallucinogen-related perceptual symptoms; American Psychiatric Association, 2013a).

Stimulants. Cocaine and methamphetamine are stimulants—meaning they enhance activity in the central nervous system. Stimulants create a sense of euphoria, with the fastest administration routes being smoking and injecting, whereas snorting has a slower onset of euphoria but a longer euphoric episode (National Institute on Drug Abuse, 2013, 2016). In addition to euphoria, stimulants may be used for the purpose of losing weight, increasing energy, and improving attention and concentration. Stimulant use can lead to acute medical problems, such as heart arrhythmia and attacks, seizures and strokes, and death. Paranoia, disorganized thinking, mood swings, and aggressive behavior may occur.

Inhalants. Inhalants cover a variety of different substances that produce vapors that can be inhaled and used in harmful ways (National Institute on Drug Abuse, 2012a). Inhaling these substances results in rapid absorption into the bloodstream, leading to quick but short-lasting euphoric effects. The effects of inhalants most closely resemble those of alcohol intoxication. Inhalants are extremely toxic and can lead to significant impairment in cognitive functioning, neurological problems, and death. The acute effects of intoxication (Humeniuk, Henry-Edwards, Ali, Poznyak, & Monteiro, 2010a) can include dizziness, drowsiness, disorientation, blurred vision, poor coordination, gastrointestinal problems (nausea and vomiting, ulcers, diarrhea), and unpredictable behavior. These effects increase the risk of accidents and injuries resulting from use.

Over-the-Counter Drugs

In addition to alcohol and illicit street drugs, some over-the-counter medications can be used in harmful ways. Dextromethorphan is a cough suppressant that creates a dissociative hallucinogenic effect (Conca & Worthen, 2012). Caffeine is a stimulant consumed by most children and adults on a regular basis. While the *DSM–5* does not recognize a caffeine use disorder, it does recognize caffeine intoxication, withdrawal, and caffeine-induced disorders. Excessive caffeine consumption can result in nausea, vomiting, abdominal pain, diarrhea, headache, insomnia, agitation, tremor, abnormally high muscle tension, tinnitus, elevated heart rate, and delirium (Conca & Worthen, 2012). Caffeine, particularly in energy drinks, is also mixed with alcohol to counteract the sedative effects of alcohol, making users subjectively feel less intoxicated and maintaining desire to continue drinking (Heinz, de Wit, Lilje, & Kassel, 2013). While newer antihistamines (e.g., loratadine, cetirizine) are not often associated with misuse, older ones such as diphenhydramine, pheniramine, and cyclizine are often implicated in misuse (Conca & Worthen, 2012).

Prescription Drugs

Whereas all illegal drugs are designated as Schedule I substances by the Drug Enforcement Agency, indicating that they have high potential for harmful use and no established medical use in the United States (e.g., heroin, gamma-hydroxybutyrate), drugs that have scientifically established medical use but also have potential for harmful use are designated Schedule II to V based on the potential for harmful use and public health risk tied to each substance (Drug Enforcement Agency, 2017). Lower numbers indicate increasing abuse potential and decreasing legal access than higher numbers, so drugs such as morphine and cocaine are Schedule II, whereas cough medicines with codeine are Schedule V. In Chapters 6 and 7, we discuss implications for treatment of anxiety and sleep problems in patients with co-occurring harmful substance use, given that some of the most widely prescribed medications for anxiety and sleep are Schedule IV drugs.

Detecting and understanding harmful use of prescription medications is more complex than with illicit drugs because often these medications are originally prescribed for legitimate medical conditions and the typical transition from appropriate medication use to a drug use disorder can be gradual. There are a variety of somewhat contradictory definitions for various types of inappropriate use of prescription drugs (Zacny et al., 2003). According to the National Institute on Drug Abuse (2018c), prescription drug misuse means "taking a medication in a manner or dose other than prescribed; taking someone else's prescription, even if for a legitimate medical complaint such as pain; or taking a medication to feel euphoria (i.e., to get high)" (p. 3).

The most commonly abused prescription medications include opioid analgesics (i.e., pain medications such as Percocet [oxycodone/acetaminophen] or Norco [hydrocodone/acetaminophen]), benzodiazepines (i.e., antianxiety medications such as Xanax [alprazolam] and Valium [diazepam]), sleep aids that are similar chemically to benzodiazepines (e.g., Ambien [zolpidem]), and stimulants (i.e., ADHD medications such as Adderall [dextroamphetamine/amphetamine]). Problems related to misuse of opioids have gained national attention as rates of opioid overdose deaths have grown significantly, with 46 individuals dying every day due to pre-scription opioid overdoses (Hedegaard, Warner, & Miniño, 2017). About 85% of treatment-seeking heroin users began opioid use with a prescrip-tion opioid (Cicero, Ellis, Surratt, & Kurtz, 2014). Opioids disproportion-ately account for the highest number of deaths due to risks for respiratory depression, particularly when samples are tainted with extremely power-ful opioids such as fentanyl and carfentanyl. The acute effects of opioid misuse include nausea and vomiting, drowsiness, poor memory and con-centration, and reduced sexual functioning. Misuse of prescription opioids frequently results in financial difficulties and criminal behavior to obtain opioids.

Sedatives, such as benzodiazepines and sleep aids, are prescribed as anti-anxiety and sleep medications, as well as for seizures, muscle pain, and surgical procedures (Humeniuk et al., 2010a). These medications can quickly lead to tolerance and extremely aversive withdrawal syndromes. When combined with alcohol, opioids, or other respiratory depressants, the risk of death from overdose rises significantly. The acute effects of mis-use include drowsiness and confusion, poor memory and concentration, and poor coordination.

Prescription stimulants are generally prescribed for attention-deficit/hyperactivity disorder and include drugs such as Adderall [dextroamphet-amine/amphetamine], Ritalin [methylphenidate], and Concerta [methyl-phenidate] (National Institute on Drug Abuse, 2018a). These drugs are sometimes misused by students to improve performance on exams or reduce need for sleep. They also may be misused as diet aids. Crushing the pills to snort or inject can lead to intense euphoric reactions and increased alertness and energy, similar to illicit stimulants such as cocaine. Health-related problems are similar as well, including heart arrhythmia and fail-ure, seizures, paranoia, and psychotic symptoms.

SUMMARY

Alcohol and drug use occur on a continuum. Given how common drinking and drug use are, it is important for psychologists and other mental health professionals to be able to identify whether a patient's use of alcohol and drugs is placing them at risk, already causing problems, or needs specialized treatments. Some patients stay within low-risk or moderate drinking guidelines and do not take any medications or have medical conditions that contraindicate alcohol use. Others are not yet having any significant problems but are using alcohol or drugs in ways that are risky or hazardous. Still others are using in ways that have begun to cause problems ranging from mild and infrequent to severe and recurrent and may need specialty care. The next three chapters provide further guidance on how and why harmful substance use develops, how to determine what type of treatment a patient needs, and how to talk to patients about their alcohol and drug use.

2

ETIOLOGY AND SOCIOCULTURAL ASPECTS OF HARMFUL SUBSTANCE USE

Addressing harmful substance use requires some understanding of the factors that lead to the initiation, maintenance, and escalation of this behavior. An important starting point in this understanding is knowledge of the epidemiology of harmful substance use in the general population, in specific medical populations, and in vulnerable or health disparate populations. As reviewed in this chapter, harmful substance use is common and may be increasing in the United States. Part of the explanation for harmful substance use lies within the chemical properties of the substances themselves and the impact they have on the human brain, so the chapter provides a brief overview of neurobiological models of addiction. However, consistent with the focus of psychology on learning experiences, emotions, and environment as influences of behavior, the chapter also discusses how these factors may contribute to harmful substance use generally and in specific medical and vulnerable or health disparate populations.

http://dx.doi.org/10.1037/0000160-003
Psychological Treatment of Medical Patients Struggling With Harmful Substance Use,
by J. A. Schumacher and D. C. Williams

EPIDEMIOLOGY

Much of what is known about the prevalence and correlates of harmful alcohol and drug use in the U.S. population comes from two large epidemiological surveys. The National Epidemiologic Survey on Alcohol and Related Conditions (NESARC) is a psychiatric epidemiological survey that included three waves of data collection (2001–2002, 2004–2005, and 2012–2103; Hasin & Grant, 2015). The National Survey on Drug Use and Health (NSDUH) began in 1971 and is conducted every year in all 50 states and Washington, DC, under the direction of the Substance Abuse and Mental Health Services Administration (SAMHSA, 2017; see also Center for Behavioral Health Statistics and Quality, 2016). Thus, between these two sources, a great deal is known about epidemiology and trends in alcohol and drug use in the United States. We outline some recent key findings next.

Alcohol

Alcohol is the most widely used substance in the United States, so it is not surprising that alcohol use disorders are the most common substance use disorders (SAMHSA, 2017). Estimates from NESARC-III indicate that the 12-month prevalence of *DSM–5* alcohol use disorder was 13.9% and the lifetime prevalence was 29.1% (American Psychiatric Association, 2013a; Grant et al., 2015). Binge drinking is also common in adults, with about 27% of individuals 18 years old and older self-reporting binge drinking in the last month. While binge drinking occurs across the lifespan, it is most common in 18- to 25-year-olds and occurs more commonly in men than women (Center for Behavioral Health Statistics and Quality, 2016).

Illicit Drugs

Illicit drug use is also highest in the 18- to 25-year-old age category, in which 23.2% of individuals have used in the past month (SAMHSA, 2017). According to the 2015 NSDUH, the mostly commonly used illicit drug is cannabis, with 24 million Americans age 12 or older reporting current use (Center for Behavioral Health Statistics and Quality, 2016). Cannabis use disorder was the most commonly reported drug use disorder in NESARC-III, reported by approximately 2.5% of the U.S. population (Grant et al., 2016). Following marijuana, hallucinogens were the most commonly tried illicit drugs (15.3%); cocaine and methamphetamine use were reported by 14.5% and 5.4%, respectively; and inhalant use had a lifetime prevalence of 9.6% in the 2015 NSDUH (Center for Behavioral Health Statistics and Quality, 2016). Estimates from NESARC-III indicate that 4% of U.S. adults met *DSM–5* diagnostic criteria for a past year drug use disorder (2% mild and 2% moderate or severe) and 10% met lifetime criteria (Grant et al., 2015).

Prescription Medications

Misuse of prescription medications is common, with 7.1% of people age 12 or older misusing a prescription medication in the past year and 4.7% specifically misusing prescription opioids (Center for Behavioral Health Statistics and Quality, 2016). According to NESARC-III, in 2012–2013 an estimated 1% of the population met criteria for an opioid use disorder (Grant et al., 2016). Prescription medication misuse occurs across the developmental continuum. Between 2002–2003 and 2012–2013, rates of lifetime nonmedical use of prescription opioids, tranquilizers, and stimulants increased for adults over the age of 50 (Schepis & McCabe, 2016), a population that tends to have more medical comorbidities and may be more susceptible to drug–drug interactions or other adverse effects. At the other end of the spectrum, adolescents, who may also be more vulnerable to medication effects, also report high lifetime rates of nonmedical use of prescription drugs (McCabe & West, 2013, 2014; McCabe, West, Teter, & Boyd, 2012).

Trends

As shown in Table 2.1, comparison of data from NESARC-I and NESARC-III suggests that harmful substance use may be on the rise (Grant et al., 2017; Hasin et al., 2015; Martins et al., 2017; Saha et al., 2016).

TABLE 2.1. Trends in Alcohol and Drug Use/Disorder from 2001-2002 to 2012-2013

Disorder	2001-2002	2012-2013
High-risk drinking/alcohol use disorder	9.7%/8.5%	12.6%/12.7%
Marijuana use/use disorder	4.1%/1.5%	9.5%/2.9%
Heroin use/use disorder	0.3%/1.6%	0.2%/0.7%
Prescription opioid misuse/use disorder	1.8%/0.4%	4.1%/0.8%

Note. Data from Grant et al. (2017), Hasin et al. (2015), Martins et al. (2017), and Saha et al. (2016).

HARMFUL SUBSTANCE USE AMONG PATIENTS IN MEDICAL SETTINGS

Psychologists working with medical patients should have an idea of how common harmful substance use may be in the specific patient populations with which they work as well as the unique impacts harmful substance use may have on these patients. People with substance use disorders often have one or more accompanying medical issues: lung or cardiovascular disease, stroke, cancer, or psychiatric disorders (National Institute on Drug Abuse, 2014). Many effects relate to long-term use (e.g., marijuana and lung disease; alcohol use and cancer). In addition, drugs such as inhalants have neurotoxic effects that may cause serious harm with use of shorter duration. Alcohol can compromise immune function, which may increase vulnerability to illness when exposed to infectious diseases. Intravenous use of drugs such as heroin, methamphetamine, and cocaine is also linked to increased risk for infectious disease, accounting for 9% of HIV diagnoses in 2016. Next, we focus specifically on primary care, cancer, cardiac, and women's health settings as typical settings where clinical health psychologists may work.

Primary Care Treatment Settings

When universal screening for alcohol and drug use is implemented in primary care settings, evidence from one study suggests that almost one quarter of patients will report exceeding low-risk guidelines for alcohol use or engaging in drug use (Madras et al., 2009). Consistent with epidemiological research, the most commonly reported harmful substance use was alcohol, with 42.1% of patients screening positive reporting heavy alcohol use and 15.5% reporting marijuana use. Smaller numbers reported using cocaine, heroin, methamphetamines, or other drugs. Focusing specifically on alcohol use in family medicine patients, another study found that approximately 22% of men and 6.5% of women scored above the low-risk cut-off on a widely used alcohol screening tool developed by the World Health Organization (Rubinsky, Kivlahan, Volk, Maynard, & Bradley, 2010).

Alcohol is known to negatively affect several medical conditions commonly treated in primary care settings. For example, one research study showed increasing levels of poor adherence to diabetic treatment with increasing levels of alcohol use, with adherence-related problems starting with even one drink per day (Ahmed, Karter, & Liu, 2006). A meta-analysis of the connection between alcohol use and risk of hypertension found an increased risk of hypertension with any alcohol consumption in men and drinking more than one to two drinks per day in women (Roerecke et al., 2018). Although moderate alcohol use may have some beneficial effects on the immune system, chronic heavy alcohol use has broad deleterious effects on immune functioning, which may increase risk for infections and cancer as well as impairing response to vaccinations (Pasala, Barr, & Messaoudi, 2015).

Cancer Treatment Settings

Although risk for misuse is often given less consideration in prescribing opioids to cancer patients, there is evidence that this may be an at-risk population. In a study of the insurance claims for almost 40,000 patients who filled an opioid prescription following curative-intent surgery for one of several forms of cancer, more than 10% refilled at least one prescription 90 to 180 days later. This is considered persistent opioid use. This study was important because it focused specifically on patients who had not filled an opioid prescription in more than a year prior to the surgery (Lee et al., 2017). Although this pattern of opioid use is not indicative of opioid misuse or an opioid use disorder, persistent opioid use is associated with increased risk for opioid use disorder in patients with chronic noncancer pain (Dowell, Haegerich, & Chou, 2016). Evidence for this risk in cancer patients comes from work such as a one-month retrospective chart review study of cancer patients in a palliative care clinic in 2012 (Barclay, Owens, & Blackhall, 2014). Researchers found that 43% of the palliative care patients treated scored in the medium- to high-risk range on a measure of opioid risk. Although urine drug screens were available for only 40% of patients, almost half of the screens had abnormal findings. Similarly, in a survey of palliative care medicine fellowship program directors, 19 out of 38 respondents indicated that harmful substance use and diversion was a problem for their clinic (Tan, Barclay, & Blackhall, 2015). As is the case in other patient populations, harmful substance use in cancer patients is not limited to opioids. One study found that 17% of advanced cancer patients in a palliative care clinic screened positive for alcohol problems (Dev et al., 2011).

Cardiac Treatment Settings

Although alcohol has long been viewed as cardio-protective (Costanzo, Di Castelnuovo, Donati, Iacoviello, & Gaetano, 2010), recent research suggests that this may be an artifact of methodological issues in prior research.

Specifically, research demonstrating protective effects of moderate alcohol use relative to abstaining from alcohol often combined former drinkers with lifetime abstainers into a single abstainer group. However, former drinkers who currently abstain from alcohol may do so because they are in poor health, which may inflate the apparent protective effects of moderate alcohol consumption (Toma, Paré, & Leong, 2017). Although the evidence on whether drinking moderate amounts of alcohol protects heart health relative to abstaining from alcohol has been called into question, the evidence that heavy alcohol consumption (more than 14 drinks per week in women and more than 21 drinks per week in men) increases risk for mortality is much clearer (Toma et al., 2017). There is also evidence that implementing screening and brief intervention for alcohol may have positive impacts on hypertension for some patients (Chi, Weisner, Mertens, Ross, & Sterling, 2017). Smoking marijuana, which may be increasingly common in patients across health-care settings, has also been linked to increased risk for heart disease and acute coronary events (Singla, Sachdeva, & Mehta, 2012; Thomas, Kloner, & Rezkalla, 2014). Although less prevalent, use of most other illegal drugs and prescription misuse have potential to cause significant acute effects on the cardiovascular system and damage to the heart (Ghuran & Nolan, 2000).

Women's Health Treatment Settings

The lifetime prevalence of alcohol use disorders is lower in women, but this gap may be decreasing over time. Moreover, despite women's lower risk for alcohol-related problems, there is evidence for gender-based health disparities in the area of harmful substance use (Greenfield, Back, Lawson, & Brady, 2010; Greenfield et al., 2007). Substance use disorder treatment seems to be equally effective for men and women, but there is evidence that women with lifetime substance use disorders are less likely to receive substance use disorder treatment than men with lifetime substance use disorders. This may be because women face unique barriers to treatment including those related to pregnancy and child-care responsibilities, which many treatment programs are not equipped to address (Greenfield et al., 2007). There is also evidence that women may experience a faster progression from onset of harmful substance use to severe substance use disorder. Although the reasons for this "telescoping" are unclear, this may result in women entering treatment with more severe substance-related problems (Greenfield et al., 2010). Women are also more likely to experience disorders such as anxiety and depression, which may serve as a barrier to treatment entry given the lack of programs that adequately address dual disorders and may contribute to relapse after substance use disorder treatment if not addressed (Albert, 2015; Greenfield et al., 2007; McLean, Asnaani, Litz, & Hofmann, 2011).

Women's health treatment settings represent important places for alcohol screening and intervention because many women rely on these settings for primary care. These settings also address reproductive health, an area where harmful drug and alcohol use often receives the most attention. Prenatal substance use can have serious effects on infants and mothers. Opioid use during pregnancy can cause neonatal abstinence syndrome, a type of withdrawal in the newborn child. Prenatal alcohol exposure is the leading preventable cause of birth defects in the United States and there is no known amount of alcohol that is safe to consume during pregnancy (National Institute on Drug Abuse, 2014; Ondersma, Simpson, Brestan, & Ward, 2000). Pregnant women who engage in harmful substance use often have delays in entering prenatal care and are at high risk of separation from children after birth, due to child protection policies and legislation regarding illicit substance use (Marcenko, Kemp, & Larson, 2000; Pagnini & Reichman, 2000). The complexities of treating pregnant women who engage in harmful substance use are depicted in the case illustration in Chapter 8, this volume.

ETIOLOGY

An understanding of why people use, misuse, or develop substance use disorders is an important starting point for thinking about how concerned to be about a particular patient's reports of alcohol or drug use. Initiation of alcohol and drug use is typically the result of a complex interplay of genetics and sociocultural influences. The escalation and maintenance of alcohol and drug use brings a third important factor into the equation, the impact of drugs and alcohol on the brain (i.e., the neurobiology of addiction).

The Neurobiology of Addiction

Why is it that a patient using oxycodone to manage headache pain is at risk of losing control over use of the medication and developing an opioid use disorder, whereas a patient using acetaminophen to manage headache pain does not incur risk for acetaminophen use disorder? The answer lies largely in how the substances affect the brain. Only psychoactive substances—those that alter mood, perception, or cognition—lead to substance use disorder

(Black & Andreasen, 2014). In general, when it comes to harmful substance use, many people use substances to feel good; most drugs that are used in harmful ways cause intense pleasure or euphoria during intoxication (National Institute on Drug Abuse, 2014). For example, in addition to using opioids for pain relief, individuals who went on to develop opioid use disorders described feelings of euphoria or warmth when opioids were first ingested or shortly thereafter (Cicero & Ellis, 2017). However, for individuals with co-occurring psychiatric illnesses such as depression, anxiety, or trauma and stressor related disorders, harmful substance use may be an effort to feel less bad (Cicero & Ellis, 2017; National Institute on Drug Abuse, 2014). In other cases, harmful substance use is linked to the enhancement effects of the substance as in the case of nonprescribed use of stimulant medication to enhance academic performance (Teter, McCabe, LaGrange, Cranford, & Boyd, 2006).

But what about drugs like Prozac (fluoxetine hydrochloride)? Prozac, which was the most widely prescribed medication in 2007 (National Public Radio, 2007), has demonstrated impacts on mood, but patients do not develop Prozac use disorder. This brings us to the next key aspect of substances associated with their risk for being used in harmful ways, the mechanism of action in the brain. Research indicates that all drugs that can cause substance use disorders act directly or indirectly on the brain's reward system. Pathways in the brain's limbic system, particularly the pathway between the ventral tegmental area in the midbrain and the nucleus accumbens in the forebrain, are activated during drug use and other emotionally rewarding behaviors such as eating food, having sex, and socializing (Nestler, 2005). When applied to natural rewards, the reward pathways in the brain are adaptive; they help us seek out and repeat behavior likely to promote survival. When some drugs are taken they can trigger the release of two to 10 times the amount of dopamine that natural rewards do in these brain regions. Moreover, the effect can last much longer. This enhanced reward response to harmful substances can change the way the system responds to naturally rewarding behaviors. If drug use continues, other activities may become less pleasurable because the dopamine system down-regulates to deal with the excess (National Institute on Drug Abuse, 2014; Nestler, 2005).

In addition to its psychoactive effects, the speed with which a substance produces intoxication or high tends to increase the likelihood that its use will be escalated over time. As a result, routes of administration that increase how quickly a substance is absorbed into the blood, for example, crushing and snorting, rather than taking prescription opioids by mouth, typically increase the intensity of intoxication and likelihood of escalating use. Shorter-acting substances may be more likely to produce withdrawal than longer-acting substances. For example, shorter-acting benzodiazepines may be more likely to lead to development of withdrawal than longer-acting benzodiazepines. Given that desire to avoid or abate withdrawal can promote continued use, longer-acting substances, which tend to be associated with a longer but less intense withdrawal syndrome, are sometimes used to reduce risk for misuse (American Psychiatric Association, 2013a; Schaeffer, 2012).

Although the substances themselves tell part of the story, they do not tell the full story. Many patients take medications, even those with high potential for causing substance use disorders, only as prescribed and never misuse them. Many patients consume alcohol in moderation or infrequently use marijuana or other drugs recreationally and never progress to a pattern of heavier use or regular use. Thus, having knowledge of the neurobiology of addiction is necessary to understand harmful substance use, but it is not sufficient. It is important to understand other factors that explain escalation of use and development of substance use disorders. Unfortunately, another key factor that predicts harmful substance use is largely out of patients' control. It is estimated that genetic and epigenetic factors account for an average of 50% of vulnerability to substance use disorder, with the strongest evidence for alcohol use disorder (Li & Burmeister, 2009; National Institute on Drug Abuse, 2014). Harmful substance use frequently co-occurs with other mental health disorders such as anxiety and depression. Some of this co-occurrence may be explained by shared genetic liability, but there is also evidence that mental health disorders predict onset of later substance use disorders (Swendsen et al., 2010).

Sociocultural Factors and Health Disparities

Adolescence and young adulthood are high-risk times for the onset of harmful drug and alcohol use. Factors such as curiosity and peer pressure as well as perceptions that alcohol and drug use are normative by both adolescents and their caregivers may promote initiation or maintenance of use in adolescents. Environmental factors such as family members who use drugs or alcohol or engage in criminal behavior, drug-using peers, academic failure, or poor social skills can increase risk for initiation and maintenance. Earlier onset of substance use is predictive of substance use disorder (National Institute on Drug Abuse, 2014) and adolescent alcohol use—even at levels below the diagnostic threshold for a use disorder—predicts future alcohol and drug use disorders in young adulthood (Rohde, Lewinsohn, Kahler, Seeley, & Brown, 2001). In sum, although adolescence is often thought of as a time when experimentation with drugs and alcohol is normative and perhaps even benign, the data suggest that this experimentation is not benign and may lead to serious negative outcomes for some youth.

There is a unique mosaic of health disparities related to harmful alcohol and drug use in the United States. With the exception of Native Americans, racial and ethnic minorities generally have lower rates of alcohol and drug use disorders than White, non-Hispanic individuals (Grant et al., 2015, 2016). In the third wave of the NESARC, the rate of current alcohol use disorder was 19.2% for Native Americans (relative to 13.9% for White, non-Hispanic individuals) and the rate of current drug use disorder was 6.9% (relative to 3.7% for White, non-Hispanic individuals). Although they may not be at higher risk for substance use disorder, there is evidence that African Americans and Hispanics are underserved relative to Whites in the substance use disorder treatment system and come to treatment with distinct needs that may require treatment matching (Marsh, Cao, Guerrero, & Shin, 2009). Lesbian, gay, bisexual, and transgender women and men may also be at higher risk for harmful substance use and substance use disorders (Hughes & Eliason, 2002; McCabe, Hughes, Bostwick, West, & Boyd, 2009). Also, as outlined previously, women are less likely to develop substance use disorders than men, but they are also less likely to receive treatment if they do develop a substance use disorder (Greenfield et al., 2007). Lower socioeconomic status predicts greater risk for alcohol and drug use disorder as does being divorced or never married (Grant, Goldstein, et al., 2015; Grant, Saha, et al., 2016).

SUMMARY

Substance use disorders are common in the United States. It is estimated that approximately 14% of Americans have a current alcohol use disorder and approximately 4% have a current drug use disorder. Cannabis and opioids are the drugs most likely to be used in harmful ways, and there is evidence that harmful use of these two drugs and alcohol has been increasing over recent years. Given the prevalence of harmful substance use in the U.S. population, it is not surprising that medical patients in a variety of settings may have a presenting picture that is complicated by harmful substance use. Primary care is an important setting for screening and early intervention for harmful alcohol and drug use, and also is a point of entry into the treatment system for numerous acute and chronic illnesses and injuries that may be linked to harmful substance use. In cancer treatment settings, there is a delicate balance between adequate pain management and managing risk for opioid misuse. In cardiac treatment settings, chronic alcohol and drug use may increase risk for development of cardiovascular disease, and acute use of many substances may place patients at greater risk for acute cardiovascular events. Although women are less likely to develop substance use disorders than men, they are also less likely to access care for substance use disorder when they do. This combined with the unique risks tied to prenatal substance use makes women's health settings important places for intervention. Given the strong role of genetics, the neurobiological effects of alcohol and drug use, and other factors outside patient and provider control, prevention and early intervention are keys to addressing harmful substance use in medical settings. In attempting to implement these strategies, it is important for providers to be aware of unique health disparities that may make some patients more likely to develop harmful substance use and might serve as barriers to help for other patients.

3

LEVELS OF CARE AND STANDARD TREATMENTS FOR HARMFUL SUBSTANCE USE

As is reviewed further in Chapter 4, determining whether a patient's use of alcohol and drugs exceeds low-risk guidelines is a fairly straightforward task. However, knowing that a patient drinks or uses in risky ways, and even knowing that they have a use disorder, is just a starting place for determining what types of treatments and other services will be most likely to help them. Several guidelines delineate the most important elements of conducting an assessment for patients who have or are suspected to have a substance use disorder. An outline of guidelines from the American Psychiatric Association is included in this chapter. Assessment findings and patient preference play an important role in determining which treatment option is right for the patient, but two other important criteria should also guide such decisions. First, although several evidence-based treatments for substance use disorders have been developed and tested, not all facilities offer evidence-based care (Fletcher, 2013). We review evidence-based treatment options to help guide referral decisions. Second, criteria developed by the American Society for Addiction Medicine to determine which level of care is most appropriate for patients will be presented.

http://dx.doi.org/10.1037/0000160-004

Psychological Treatment of Medical Patients Struggling With Harmful Substance Use,
by J. A. Schumacher and D. C. Williams

BIOPSYCHOSOCIAL ASSESSMENT

Across substance use guidelines, there is agreement that assessments should be holistic and include elements within biological, psychological, and social domains. For readers seeking guidelines for specialized evaluation of substance use, the American Society for Addiction Medicine (ASAM) also has released comprehensive recommendations (Mee-Lee, Shulman, Fishman, Gastfriend, & Miller, 2013). While an addiction treatment program is likely to have the expertise and resources to provide such comprehensive assessments, within most medical settings provision of such assessments is not feasible. The depth of assessment of substance use will vary across medical settings depending on their needs and resources. In some settings, brief screening and referral to treatment or additional resources is adequate. This approach is explained in depth in Chapter 4. In other settings, such as integrated health settings where more significant behavioral health resources are provided, a more comprehensive evaluation may be beneficial, and brief treatment options may be available or could be developed to be provided within that setting.

While the American Psychological Association has not developed practice guidelines for substance use, a pragmatic set of recommendations is provided in the American Psychiatric Association's *Treatment of Patients with Substance Use Disorders* (2006), with seven domains of assessment: (a) history of past and present substance use, including effects on cognitive, psychological, behavioral, and physiological functioning; (b) general medical and psychiatric history and examination; (c) history of previous psychiatric treatments and outcomes; (d) family and social history; (e) screening of blood, breath, or urine for substance use; (f) other laboratory tests to confirm or rule out the presence of conditions that frequently co-occur with substance use; and (g) collateral information from significant others, with patient's consent. Psychologists and other mental health providers should collaborate with medical colleagues to obtain the medical components of the assessment when necessary. Multimodal and multiinformant assessment is the gold standard, because although self-reports of alcohol and drug use are surprisingly valid measures when compared with other sources of information, some patients may underreport their use of substances particularly in initial contacts with providers (Rockett, Putnam, Jia, & Smith, 2006; Weiss et al., 1998).

In assessing alcohol and drug use, it is important to be aware of unique legal and ethical issues that may arise. Patients expect and are legally entitled to have their privacy safeguarded and health care information kept confidential. And as Saitz (2013) noted, general health care settings have an advantage over substance use treatment settings in that regard because patients can be evaluated and receive care without being identified as engaging in harmful substance use simply by being in the setting. However, in a general health care setting, medical records might be viewed by a broader range of providers and released by patients to a broader number of entities, and records in these settings are not clearly protected by CFR 42 Part 2, a federal statute that affords extra protection for substance use treatment records. Thus, consistent with ethical standards, it is important that providers are aware of state and federal statutes and document substance use issues accurately, avoiding ambiguous or stigmatizing language that might be misunderstood by others who view the record. For example, a provider should avoid statements such as "patient reports abusing alcohol" and instead use language such as "patient reports consuming five to six standard drinks on weeknights, and 12 or more drinks on weekend days."

Patient substance use may also result in mandatory reporting, and statutes regarding such reports vary from state to state (Weaver, 2013). It is important for providers to be aware of relevant state statutes and to follow ethical mandates to make patients aware of any limits to confidentiality these statutes may impose on a particular therapeutic encounter or service and obtain proper informed consent. For example, some states require reporting of seizures to the department of motor vehicles or its equivalent, including alcohol withdrawal seizures. Because substance use affects parenting and child development, reports of substance use by parents of minor children or pregnant women as well as children or adolescents themselves may meet legal or ethical standards for a report to child protective services. As statutes vary by state, it is important for providers to be aware of whether their state has any mandatory reporting requirements related to substance use, which may require reports even in cases where a provider does not have reasonable suspicion that harm has occurred or will occur. Mandatory reporting is a feature of the clinical vignette in Chapter 8, this volume.

DIAGNOSTIC ASSESSMENT

In medical settings where more formal diagnostic assessment of criteria for substance use disorders is beneficial, valid and reliable assessment is best performed with the use of both a structured interview and self-administered assessment instruments. Having multiple points of data allows clinicians to find converging evidence to support their diagnosis. Unfortunately, the most commonly used structured interviews are based on criteria in the fourth edition of the *Diagnostic and Statistical Manual of Mental Disorders* (American Psychiatric Association, 2000), so awareness of the changes in criteria is important when administering these instruments (see the review in Chapter 1, this volume).

Self-administered assessment measures also can provide valuable information about a patient's substance use. These can be administered via paper and pencil or computer/electronic device (Khazaal et al., 2015). For alcohol, instruments such as the Alcohol Use Disorder Identification Test, Adapted for Use in the United States (USAUDIT; Babor, Higgins-Biddle, & Saunders, 2016) or the shorter version (AUDIT-C; Bush, Kivlahan, McDonell, Fihn, & Bradley, 1998) are recommended. For drugs, instruments such as the Drug Abuse Screening Test (DAST; H. A. Skinner, 1982) and the Alcohol, Smoking and Substance Involvement Screening Test (ASSIST; World Health Organization ASSIST Working Group, 2002) are commonly used. The National Institute on Alcohol Abuse and Alcoholism (2003) provides a useful guide to tools for assessing alcohol problems including information about ordering. Tools for assessing alcohol and drug use can be obtained from the World Health Organization (https://www.who.int/substance_abuse/publications/en/), the National Institute on Drug Abuse (https://www.drugabuse.gov/nidamed-medical-health-professionals/tool-resources-your-practice/screening-assessment-drug-testing-resources/chart-evidence-based-screening-tools), and the National Institute on Alcohol Abuse and Alcoholism (https://pubs.niaaa.nih.gov/publications/assessingalcohol/index.htm).

Using self-administered measures in addition to interviews may increase patients' willingness to disclose substance use (Rosen, Henson, Finney, & Moos, 2000). Moreover, these measures can be used in addition to diagnostic information to get a sense of the severity of a patient's substance use and related problems. For example, the manual for the USAUDIT contains cut scores that can be used to inform decisions about whether to refer a patient to treatment and what level of treatment might be most appropriate (Babor et al., 2016). Norms from these measures can also serve as a basis for providing feedback to patients about their substance use using interventions such as motivational enhancement therapy (Miller, Zweben, DiClemente, & Rychtarik, 1999).

TREATMENTS FOR SUBSTANCE USE DISORDERS

While substance use disorders tend to be chronic and may include episodes of returning to use, there are a variety of evidence-based treatments for addiction, including both psychotherapies and pharmacotherapies, that may enhance outcomes. It is important to note that there can be multiple roads to recovery, and not every treatment will work for every patient. As with prescription medications, if one approach does not produce significant benefit, another evidence-based treatment should be tried.

Psychotherapeutic Treatments for Medical Settings

Motivational interviewing (MI; Miller & Rollnick, 2013) is designed to decrease patients' ambivalence about changing their substance use, increase their confidence in their own abilities to effectively make change, and create plans for how best to make the changes they desire. Treatment could be as brief as a single session or could include multiple encounters.

Motivational enhancement therapy (MET; Miller, Zweben, DiClemente, & Rychtarik, 1999) is a manualized version of MI that is developed to be four sessions in length. It includes providing feedback to patients, comparing their own use to others in the population as a way of increasing their motivation to change. It is a brief intervention with outcomes similar to those of longer treatments such as cognitive behavior therapy (CBT). Due to their brief nature, MI and MET are recommended for implementation into medical settings where integrated behavioral services are supported.

Specialized Psychotherapeutic Treatments for Specialty Settings

Several psychotherapies have been shown to be effective in treating addiction, including CBT, 12-step facilitation, behavioral couples therapy, and contingency management (National Institute on Drug Abuse, 2018b).

Cognitive Behavioral Therapy

CBT (Kadden et al., 2003) focuses on changing thinking patterns and behavior related to addiction. High-risk situations that could lead to substance use are identified, and skills are taught to decrease the likelihood of use, such as avoiding people and places where one previously used, assertively communicating to effectively refuse substances, and improving problem-solving abilities.

Twelve-Step Facilitation

Twelve-step facilitation (Nowinski, Baker, & Carroll, 1999) is a treatment designed to help patients effectively take advantage of the widely available 12-step model found in Alcoholics Anonymous or Narcotics Anonymous. While this treatment does not direct a patient through each of the steps, it teaches the patient to understand the process of engaging in 12-step programs, understand the terminology and key concepts, address barriers to attending community meetings, and do 12-step activities such as find a sponsor or identify community meetings.

Behavioral Couples Therapy

Behavioral couples therapy (McCrady & Epstein, 2009) is for couples seeking treatment for alcohol- or drug-related problems with the goals of improving the relationship functioning in addition to supporting abstinence. This treatment uses the relationship to reward healthy behaviors related to substance use and uses techniques to improve communication and increase positive activities between the partners. The use of community self-help meetings and urine drug screens is encouraged and rewarded within the context of the relationship.

Contingency Management

Contingency management (see Petry, 2000, for implementation guide) uses motivational incentives to shape patients' behavior. In this system, patients can earn incentives by engaging in desired behaviors, such as attending sessions, and having negative drug screens or alcohol breath tests. A variety of incentives can be used, including pragmatic items such as socks or bus passes, gift cards, or other desirable items such as mp3 players. While contingency management is not a traditional therapeutic approach, it is provided within the context of a therapeutic relationship with a trained provider and requires psychotherapeutic skill and expertise. The evidence is strongest for contingency management with stimulant use disorders.

Pharmacological Treatments

The U.S. Food and Drug Administration (FDA) has approved medications for the treatment of alcohol and opioid use disorders. These medications are generally intended to be used in combination with psychological treatment rather than as stand-alone treatments. Unfortunately, there are not currently medications approved for the treatment of any other substance use disorders. Historically, pharmacotherapy for substance use disorders has been underutilized and, unfortunately, is often not provided in community substance use disorder treatment programs (National Institute on Drug Abuse, 2018b). Ideally, pharmacotherapy options would be available in primary care and integrated behavioral health settings. While psychologists in most states do not have prescribing authority, psychologists and other behavioral health providers can play an important role in helping patients understand that pharmacotherapies can play an important role in their treatment. Developing collaborative relationships with medical providers will allow psychologists to more effectively assist patients with receiving comprehensive care. While psychologists should always work within their own competencies, at times they may be in a position to help medical providers be aware of all pharmacological treatments available.

Alcohol Pharmacotherapy

Three medications—disulfiram, acamprosate, and naltrexone—are approved for the treatment of alcohol use disorder (see Kranzler & Soyka, 2018, for a recent review). Perhaps the most well-known is Antabuse (disulfiram), which works by disrupting the metabolism of alcohol in the liver, resulting in an aversive physiological reaction. Common physical symptoms include flushing, sweating, nausea and vomiting, headache, blurred vision, shortness of breath, heart palpitations, and dizziness. Severe reactions to significant alcohol consumption include severe chest pain, slow heart rate, seizure, shallow breathing, or even death. The effectiveness of Antabuse is based on the expectation that drinking would create these unpleasant symptoms and thus would not be expected to work without knowledge of the consequences of drinking. It is most effective when administered closely for adherence (M. D. Skinner, Lahmek, Pham, & Aubin, 2014).

Acamprosate (Campral) regulates glutamatergic activity in the brain, reducing symptoms of prolonged alcohol withdrawal (Donoghue et al., 2015). It is administered at abstinence; thus, patients must be able to achieve a degree of baseline abstinence for initiation. On major advantage of Acamprosate is that it is not metabolized through the liver. As a result, patients who have increased liver enzymes due to drinking may still be appropriate for this medication. Disadvantages include dosing that is three times per day and a small increase in the potential for suicidal ideation or worsened depression.

Naltrexone is a synthetic opioid antagonist that blocks the opioid receptors that are involved in the reinforcing effects of alcohol thought to maintain continued use of alcohol and craving for alcohol during periods of abstinence (Volpicelli, Watson, King, Sherman, & O'Brien, 1995). It comes in both an oral and an injectable formulation. Oral dosing is daily, while the injectable version is administered once a month. The availability of once a month dosing is a major advantage for patients who struggle with adherence to medication regimens. Naltrexone is generally contraindicated for those with highly elevated liver enzymes.

Other medications under study, but not approved by the FDA for alcohol use disorder, include topiramate, gabapentin, and baclofen.

Opioid Pharmacotherapy

Three medications are approved by the FDA for opioid use disorder. Methadone is a synthetic opioid agonist, meaning that it provides analgesic effects and reduces cravings for opioids. Methadone has a long half-life and, as a result, can be dosed once per day. Methadone as prescribed for opioid use disorders can only be prescribed in approved opioid treatment centers. Participation requires being able to initially attend near daily visits for methadone administration, with take-home doses gradually earned based on adherence to treatment. Patients develop physiological dependence to methadone and must be weaned off slowly to avoid abrupt withdrawal symptoms.

Buprenorphine is a partial agonist; it provides partial analgesic effects in addition to reducing cravings for opioids. Some formulations also include the drug naloxone, which helps to prevent diversion or misuse by initiating withdrawal symptoms when used by injection. An advantage of buprenorphine is that it can be administered on an outpatient basis, without needing to attend a specialized opioid treatment program. As a result, it could be prescribed in a variety of settings, including emergency departments, primary care clinics, and mental health centers. Prescribers must have a special "X" waiver as part of their Drug Enforcement Agency (DEA) certification, and there are limitations to the number of patients that a prescriber can treat at one time. Nurse practitioners and physician assistants now can prescribe buprenorphine with a supervising physician who has the X waiver. Being aware of the local resources for opioid treatment programs, and developing collaborative relationships, will greatly enhance psychologists' ability to effectively refer patients to appropriate care.

Naltrexone, approved for alcohol, is also approved for opioids. It is a synthetic opioid antagonist, meaning that it blocks opioids from binding to receptors in the reward system in the brain, thereby preventing the user from getting high. As with alcohol, this medication is believed to help reduce substance use and craving over time, because users know they cannot get high if they use and if they do use despite this knowledge, they do not feel euphoric, so the use is not reinforced. As for alcohol, the monthly injection often helps patients better adhere to their medication.

Mutual-Help Resources

A variety of mutual-help resources are available to individuals interested in addressing substance use (see Chapter 9, this volume, for additional information). The most widely available is Alcoholics Anonymous and its sister organizations, such as Narcotics Anonymous. These types of groups began to appear in the 1930s to address a lack of available treatment options for individuals who were struggling with alcohol and drug use and have grown and broadened in the decades since (Henninger & Sung, 2013). Today, these are worldwide organizations with meetings available in most communities, including many rural locations. Meetings are based on the 12 steps and have a strong spiritual emphasis with a connection to a "higher power." Other self-help resources include organizations such as Rational Recovery, which applies a rational emotive behavior therapy approach to substance use and provides both in-person and online support resources.

PATIENT PLACEMENT GUIDELINES FOR SUBSTANCE USE

The American Society for Addiction Medicine (ASAM) has created guidelines for assessing for addiction as well as for matching appropriate treatments to patients based on the severity of their addiction problem. ASAM originally created guidelines in 1996, updated them in 2001, and most recently updated them according to the most recent edition of the *Diagnostic and Statistical Manual* (American Psychiatric Association, 2013a). ASAM also has created guidelines about using pharmacotherapies for alcohol use disorders (Fishman, Shulman, Mee-Lee, Kolodner, & Wilford, 2010).

The focus of the ASAM criteria (Mee-Lee et al., 2013) is to move beyond thinking of addiction as a single dimension and think holistically and multidimensionally. They have built their assessment process around six dimensions: (a) acute intoxication and/or withdrawal potential; (b) biomedical conditions and complications; (c) emotional, behavioral, or cognitive conditions and complications; (d) readiness to change; (e) relapse, continued use, or continued problem potential; and (f) recovery living environment. These dimensions are evaluated holistically to determine the most appropriate, individualized level of care for each patient.

Acute Intoxication and/or Withdrawal Potential

Some patients will present to a medical setting under the effects of a substance or even intoxicated. The first priority is to assure that any risks associated with acute intoxication are addressed. For example, intoxication on some medications such as opioids can result in respiratory depression or even death. Obtaining a medical evaluation as quickly as possible may be necessary, and it is also important that a patient with acute substance impairment is not allowed to drive, so alternate transportation should be arranged (Weaver, 2013). In addition to intoxication, many substances have well-established withdrawal syndromes. Alcohol, for example, can result not only in unpleasant physical symptoms, such as nausea, sweating, and shaking, but can also result in a serious medical condition called delirium tremens, which can be life threatening. Being able to assess for intoxication and withdrawal potential and helping patients obtain the medical treatment necessary for safe and comfortable transition off of substances is vitally important. Even outside of serious medical complications, experiencing withdrawal symptoms is unpleasant and is a common reason for patients to continue to use substances even when they desire to stop. Medications are available that can help to ease these symptoms and increase the likelihood that a patient will consider additional treatment options.

Be aware that when referring patients to addiction treatment centers, many are likely to ask about the potential for the patient to first need detoxification due to risk of withdrawal. Assessing for withdrawal risk and collaborating with medical colleagues to assist with withdrawal management will help you more effectively place patients into treatment.

Biomedical Conditions and Complications

It is common for patients with addiction to also experience acute or chronic medical conditions that can affect their treatment. Infectious diseases such as hepatitis, HIV/AIDS, and sexually transmitted infections may need to be addressed and managed. Chronic conditions such as hypertension and diabetes may need to be stabilized for a patient to safely engage in addiction treatment. For women, pregnancy will influence which pharmacotherapies are appropriate for treatment.

Emotional, Behavioral, or Cognitive Conditions or Complications

As discussed more fully in Chapters 5 and 6, "dual diagnoses"—having both an addictive disorder as well as one or more psychiatric disorders—are incredibly common. Assessing and addressing these co-occurring disorders is critically important. Treating addictive disorders and not addressing co-occurring disorders will reduce the likelihood of successful treatment and is a missed opportunity to help reduce suffering in our patients. For example, trauma-related problems are particularly prevalent in addictions, and research completed within our research group has shown that trauma treatment can be safely and effectively provided in the context of addiction treatment (Coffey et al., 2016). Some behavioral, emotional, or cognitive symptoms may be due to the effects of substances, while others may reveal a co-occurring disorder. Distinguishing between substance-induced symptoms and co-occurring psychiatric disorders is an important skill that can change the course of treatment. For example, stabilizing and managing symptoms of bipolar disorder will be necessary for effective addiction treatment.

Readiness to Change

Readiness to change is the degree to which a patient is ready or willing to engage in the recovery process. This concept is based on the "stages of change" transtheoretical model (Prochaska, DiClemente, & Norcross, 1992), which recognizes that patients are at varying levels of readiness to engage in health-related behaviors. Readiness to change varies not only across people but within a person as well. For example, a patient may have significant concerns about their illicit use of opioids but be less concerned about their use of marijuana. Similarly, a patient may be quite concerned about their unmanaged diabetes but less concerned about their use of alcohol. Individuals who are on the lower end of readiness to change would benefit from services designed to enhance motivation (e.g., motivational interviewing or motivational enhancement therapy), and services should be tailored to meet patients where they are, as opposed to trying to force patients into services for which they are not ready or in which they are not interested. For example, some patients would likely benefit from intensive addiction services based on the severity of their addiction-related problems but are not interested in engaging in intensive services. Matching the intensity of the treatment, with services in which they are interested in engaging, is much more likely to be successful.

Relapse, Continued Use, or Continued Problem Potential

This dimension assesses for the degree to which the patient is at risk to continue harmful substance use or return to problematic use. For patients with addiction histories, this assesses previous periods of reduced use or abstinence, coping skills to address use, understanding and awareness of high-risk situations and triggers to use, medications previously helpful in managing addiction, or co-occurring psychiatric and/or physical problems.

Recovery/Living Environment

Social and physical environments play key roles in either facilitating or discouraging ongoing recovery from substance use and other co-occurring situations. Family members, roommates, neighborhoods, employment, child care, legal challenges, and transportation are all important factors that can either increase or reduce the likelihood of recovery. Some environmental factors may support some aspects of recovery, but not others. For example, a family with a history of addiction may support abstinence and engagement in community 12-step meetings but not understand the availability of pharmacotherapy to address addiction.

When discussing substance use treatment options with patients, they are likely to think that "going to rehab" means attending a residential or inpatient treatment program. It is important to clarify with patients that there are multiple options for getting the right services, including several levels of outpatient treatment. Taking the time to help patients understand their options, and the importance of finding a program that meets their needs, can make the critical difference in helping a patient enter into treatment.

LEVELS OF CARE

The multidimensional assessment is used to determine which level of care would be most appropriate for the patient. While not all levels of care are available in a timely manner depending on geographic and resource limitations, prevalent levels of care are presented here, in order of least intensive to most.

Early Intervention

Early intervention services are for individuals who are at risk of developing a substance-related problem. These services include performing screening, brief intervention, and referral to treatment in a medical setting or a non-addiction setting. These approaches are covered in greater detail in the next chapter.

Outpatient Services

Services at this level are provided on an outpatient basis, focused less on intensity of services and more on meeting patients where they are. This includes individuals who would be referred to more intensive levels of treatment if their level of readiness to change were higher. As a result, these treatment settings provide motivation-enhancing treatments (e.g., motivational interviewing/enhancement therapy) as well as other psychosocial, evidence-based treatments. These services can be provided across a variety of settings, from general medical clinics, to mental health centers, to addiction treatment facilities. Services also should integrate medical and psychiatric treatments to address these co-occurring conditions. These outpatient services are also appropriate for individuals who have completed a more intensive level of treatment to provide ongoing monitoring and support. Outpatient treatment also includes medication assisted treatment programs, where patients receive pharmacotherapy for alcohol or opioid use disorders as well as additional psychosocial services to address addiction and co-occurring disorders. Outpatient services are also used as a transition for patients completing residential or intensive outpatient treatment programs.

Intensive Outpatient/Partial Hospitalization Services

While still provided on an outpatient basis, these services are more intensive and suited to address the complex needs of patients with co-occurring addiction and psychiatric or medical conditions. These programs generally occur for at least several hours, multiple days per week. Often programs offer evening programming to accommodate those who work during the day or have other limitations to their schedule. Providing or referring to address medical and psychiatric consultation, pharmacotherapy for addiction, and crisis services should be available. These programs generally have patients each assigned to an individual counselor, who creates a collaborative treatment plan. Group therapy is usually the most common form of treatment. Intensive outpatient programs also are used as a form of stepped care, with patients transitioning downward from residential treatment.

Residential/Inpatient Services

Residential and inpatient treatment programs provide care on a 24-hour basis. While there are varying degrees of intensity available with residential and inpatient treatment programs, the hallmark is that they provide a safe, secure recovery environment for those who need stabilization and development of recovery skills, outside of real-world environments where the risk to recovery may be high. Treatment within this setting generally is followed by continuing services at a lower level of treatment to promote ongoing recovery. Patients generally are assigned an individual counselor with whom they develop a treatment plan to address goals and objectives during the treatment episode. Group therapy is the most common form of treatment. In addition to psychotherapeutic interventions, adjunctive activities such as exercise, crafts and other recreational activities, and spiritual engagement are frequently provided.

Medically Managed Intensive Services

The highest intensity of care, these programs provide a 24-hour medically staffed acute care setting designed to address the addiction, co-occurring psychiatric, and physical health conditions of the most complex patients. These programs often can provide both withdrawal management as well as addiction treatment services in a comprehensive manner.

SUMMARY

Helping medical patients who are experiencing drug- or alcohol-related problems begins with a thorough biopsychosocial assessment. A thorough assessment helps identify patient strengths, weaknesses, preferences, and unique circumstances that may influence treatment decisions. Supplementing semistructured evaluations with structured interviews and self-administered assessments can enhance the clinical picture and further inform treatment decisions. Finally, knowledge of established guidelines for recommended levels of care and evidence-based treatments can help ensure that patients get the types of care that are most likely to help them achieve desired substance use outcomes.

4

ASSESSMENT AND BRIEF INTERVENTION FOR HARMFUL SUBSTANCE USE IN THE MEDICAL SETTING

Psychologists and other professionals working in mental health settings routinely provide screening for alcohol and drug use disorders, as well as referral to treatment for these disorders. However, many patients who are using alcohol or drugs in risky ways need brief interventions, but they do not necessarily need specialty substance use disorder treatment. Many psychologists and mental health professionals are not comfortable providing such brief intervention and thus either fail to adequate address risky alcohol and drug use or refer patients to an excessive level of care to address their issues. Therefore, an important gap exists in the care psychologists provide in traditional mental health settings. However, even if that gap in mental health treatment settings is filled, a much more problematic gap remains: The majority of patients with alcohol- or drug-related problems are not in mental health treatment.

Drawing heavily on our work implementing screening, brief intervention, and referral to treatment (SBIRT) in multiple clinical settings, as well as the medical school curriculum at the University of Mississippi Medical Center, the emphasis of this chapter is on providing technical and

http://dx.doi.org/10.1037/0000160-005
Psychological Treatment of Medical Patients Struggling With Harmful Substance Use,
by J. A. Schumacher and D. C. Williams

practical information necessary to disseminate this practice throughout medical settings. As discussed in Chapter 2, there are many medical settings where patients who have a substance use disorder, or whose use places them at elevated risk for developing one, can be identified and brief intervention or referral can be offered. Clinical health psychologists are necessary key stakeholders in this process, working with medical colleagues toward implementation.

There is broad agreement on the importance of universal screening for substance use in medical settings. Groups as diverse as the U.S. Preventive Services Task Force (Moyer & U.S. Preventive Services Task Force, 2013), the American Academy of Family Physicians (2017), the American Academy of Pediatrics (Levy, Williams, & American Academy of Pediatrics Committee on Substance Use and Prevention, 2016), the American College of Obstetricians and Gynecologists (2011), the Veterans Affairs/Department of Defense (2015), and the World Health Organization (Humeniuk, Henry-Edwards, Ali, Poznyak, & Monteiro, 2010a) all recommend screening for alcohol misuse (see Table 4.1 for a summary of recommendations).

TABLE 4.1. Recommended Practice Guidelines for Screening for Substance Use

Organization/agency	Recommendation
U.S. Preventive Services Task Force	In a primary care setting, screening for unhealthy alcohol use and providing brief behavioral counseling interventions for adults 18 and older (U.S. Preventive Services Task Force, 2019).
American Academy of Family Physicians	Clinicians screen adults ages 18 years or older for alcohol misuse and provide persons engaged in risky or hazardous drinking with brief alcohol counseling interventions to reduce alcohol misuse (American Academy of Family Physicians, 2017).
American Academy of Pediatrics	Pediatricians "increase their capacity in substance use detection, assessment, and intervention; and become familiar with adolescent SBIRT practices and their potential to be incorporated into universal screening and comprehensive care for adolescents in the medical home" (Levy, Williams, & American Academy of Pediatrics, 2016).
American College of Obstetricians and Gynecologists	Alcohol screening for women seeking OB-GYN care on an annual basis and within the first trimester of pregnancy (American College of Obstetricians and Gynecologists Committee on Health Care for Underserved Women, 2011).
Veterans Affairs/ Department of Defense	Screening for unhealthy alcohol use annually using the AUDIT-C or Single Item Alcohol Screening Questionnaire (SASQ; Veterans Affairs/Department of Defense, 2015).
World Health Organization	Screen all patients starting in young adulthood for unhealthy alcohol and substance use (WHO, 2010).

Universal screening for drug use does not have the same level of empirical support (Saitz et al., 2014) but can be an important tool in settings where drug use is prevalent. However, research suggests that only about half of primary care patients are screened and that these screenings often don't result in referral, guidance about cutting down, or any other intervention for patients who are drinking or using in ways that place them at risk or are harmful (Aalto, Pekuri, & Seppa, 2002; D'Amico, Paddock, Burnam, & Kung, 2005). Using clinical health psychologists as key players in SBIRT implementation has been suggested as one way to overcome barriers to screening and enhance implementation (Rahm et al., 2015).

IMPLEMENTING SBIRT

SBIRT builds on a substantial body of evidence that screening for harmful substance use, combined with brief interventions, is effective at affecting the substance use of patients receiving medical care (Babor, Del Boca, & Bray, 2017). Based on this evidence, the Substance Abuse and Mental Health Services Administration (SAMHSA) Center for Substance Abuse Treatment initiated a program in 2003 to implement SBIRT in a variety of medical settings to better integrate substance use screening and interventions into traditional medical settings, where substance use has often not been adequately addressed. Since the program began in 2003, multiple cohorts of SBIRT implementation have been completed. Additional SAMHSA grants have been provided that focused on training medical providers in SBIRT as part of educational training programs (e.g., Pringle, Kowalchuk, Meyers, & Seale, 2012).

SBIRT consists of four basic steps. The first is performing an objective screening to determine if patients are exceeding recommended guidelines for alcohol and/or drug use and to gauge the level of risk of harm related to their use. Second, objective feedback from the screening is provided to patients about their use of alcohol and drugs, as well as individualized recommendations based on the screening. Third, a brief motivational intervention is provided to patients whose use exceeds recommended guidelines. Fourth, patients whose use is already causing functional impairment are referred to appropriate treatment resources.

Screening

Screening is designed to detect health problems, or behaviors that put patients at risk for developing chronic health problems, at the earliest stage possible (Wilson & Jungner, 1968). Part of the screening process can include a brief "prescreening" designed to determine whether a patient needs a more comprehensive screening for alcohol or drugs. Prescreening is best accomplished using brief yet validated questions demonstrated to appropriately identify substance misuse. For example, the National Institute on Alcohol Abuse and Alcoholism (NIAAA) has developed a single-item question focused on identifying episodes of excessive alcohol use within the past 12 months that correctly identifies 82% of patients who misuse alcohol and correctly rules out 79% of patients who do not misuse alcohol (Smith, Schmidt, Allensworth-Davies, & Saitz, 2009). Similarly, a single-item drug screening question correctly identifies 100% of patients with drug misuse and correctly rules out 74% of patients who do not misuse drugs (Smith, Schmidt, Allensworth-Davies, & Saitz, 2010).

Additional alcohol and drug prescreening questions would include asking about average drinks per day and days of drinking per week to determine if the patient exceeds recommended daily or weekly guidelines. (See Table 4.2 for recommended prescreening questions.)

For patients whose prescreens are negative, meaning no past-year risky alcohol or drug use, the screening process is complete. For patients whose prescreen is positive, suggesting risky or harmful alcohol or drug use, there are a variety of validated yet brief screening measures for further

TABLE 4.2. Prescreening for Alcohol and Drugs

Source	Questions	Interpretation
National Institute of Alcoholism and Alcohol Abuse (Smith, Schmidt, Allensworth-Davies, & Saitz, 2009)	"How many times in the past year have you had five (men) or four (women or patients over age 65) drinks or more in a day?"	Any score of 1 or more results in administering a validated alcohol screening instrument.
Boston University Medical Center (Smith, Schmidt, Allensworth-Davies, & Saitz, 2010)	"How many times in the past year have you used an illegal drug or used a prescription medication for nonmedical reasons?"	Any score of 1 or more results in administering a validated drug screening instrument.
Two-Item Conjoint Screen for Alcohol and Other Drug Problems (R. L. Brown, Leonard, Saunders, & Papasouliotis, 2001)	1. "In the past year, have you ever drunk or used drugs more than you meant to?" 2. "Have you felt you wanted or needed to cut down on your drinking or drug use in the past year?"	Any score of 1 or more results in administering a validated alcohol or drug screening instrument.

screening. Most of these measures are publicly available at no cost. While the majority of screening instruments are specifically designed exclusively for either alcohol or drugs, the Alcohol, Smoking and Substance Involvement Screening Test (ASSIST) covers alcohol, tobacco, and drugs. Within SAMHSA's SBIRT model, the Alcohol Use Disorders Identification Test (USAUDIT) and the Drug Abuse Screening Test (DAST-10) were the most commonly used instruments. Clinicians, however, should tailor the instruments they use to their own settings and needs. See Table 4.3 for a summary of validated measures.

One key advantage of using validated screening measures is that they quickly provide valuable information about a patient's risk level related to alcohol or drugs. This information, then, is used to determine which level of intervention is most appropriate for the patient. For example, a patient who drinks more than the daily recommended guidelines a few times a year does not require the same level of intervention as a patient who has developed a severe alcohol use disorder and is likely to experience significant withdrawal symptoms if the patient decreases or stops using alcohol without appropriate medically supervised detoxification. Screening serves

TABLE 4.3. Alcohol and Drug Screening Instruments

Instrument	What does it screen for?	Additional information
Alcohol Use Disorders Identification Test (USAUDIT; Babor, Higgins-Biddle, & Saunders, 2016)	A 10-item alcohol screening instrument. Identifies risk level of alcohol use in the past year.	Developed by the World Health Organization. Tailored to U.S. drink sizes.
AUDIT-C (Alcohol Use Disorders Identification Test–Consumption; Babor et al., 2006)	A three-item alcohol screening instrument. Measures weekly alcohol consumption and excessive drinking.	Shorter version of AUDIT.
Cut down, Annoyed, Guilty, Eye-opener (CAGE)	A four-item alcohol screening instrument.	Developed by John A. Ewing (1984). This instrument lacks sensitivity to pick up on at-risk alcohol use.
Drug Abuse Screening Test (DAST-10)	A 10-item drug screening instrument. Identifies risk level for past-year drug use.	Developed by Harvey A. Skinner (1982).
Alcohol, Smoking and Substance Involvement Screening Test (ASSIST)	An eight-item alcohol and drug screening instrument.	Developed by the World Health Organization ASSIST Working Group (2002).

as a way of titrating interventions based on risk level. A second advantage of validated screening tools with established norms is that they allow clinicians to provide patients with objective information about how their use compares to other individuals, how it compares with recommended guidelines, and what kind of treatment intervention, if any, is indicated.

Successful implementation of universal SBIRT typically requires an efficient process that uses billing provider time as little as possible (Rahm et al., 2015; Vendetti et al., 2017). This requires establishment of a clinic procedure for screening patients for substance use. When possible, prescreening questions and screening instruments can be completed by patients electronically or with pencil and paper after checking in for their appointment, but before they see the provider. The clinician can then maximize their time with the patient as opposed to administering questions and instruments with their limited face-to-face time with the patient. With training, frontline staff members can effectively explain the importance and purpose of the screening to the patient. Nursing personnel can enhance efficiency by administering or reviewing prescreening or screening results to determine next steps. Establishing a process for the clinic enhances efficiency of practice. Also, using technology to assist with the screening process, such as connecting the screening instruments directly to the electronic medical record, improves the efficiency of the process and allows providers to spend their time working effectively with patients. Regardless of the procedure, having established clinic procedures and buy-in from all levels of staff members and clinicians are important lessons learned from clinics that have effectively implemented SBIRT (Hargraves et al., 2017).

Screening should include the use of biomarkers, which are medical laboratory tests that can identify biological indicators of problems due to alcohol. These biomarkers can be used in addition to self-report measures to screen for alcohol-related problems. An advantage of biomarkers is that they are not subject the limitations of self-report—mainly that people may provide information that is not accurate or may sometimes be reluctant to disclose problems. Relevant alcohol-related biomarkers include gamma-glutamyl-transferase (GGT), aspartate aminotransferase (ASAT), alanine aminotransferase (ALAT), mean corpuscular volume (MCV), and carbohydrate-deficient transferrin (CDT; Allen, Sillanaukee, Strid, & Litten, 2003). Phosphatidylethanol (PEth; Viel et al., 2012) and ethyl glucuronide (EtG; Helander, Böttcher, Fehr, Dahmen, & Beck, 2009) are commonly used for detecting heavy alcohol consumption. Depending on the setting, nonprescribing mental health clinicians may or may not have privileges to order these kinds of laboratory tests and should collaborate with their medical colleagues for laboratory testing and rely on medical expertise when interpreting these laboratory tests as well.

Urine or blood toxicology screens also can serve as objective data for identifying the presence of illicit drugs and prescription medications as well as their metabolites, which can provide indications of recent use in patients who are not currently intoxicated. In our experience, this type of adjunctive screening is common in pregnant women, patients who are seen in the emergency department, particularly if they present with cognitive or psychiatric symptoms, patients seen in pain specialty clinics, and patients in substance use treatment, but it is less common in other settings. With toxicology screens, it is extremely important to understand exactly which substances the screen is able to detect or not detect, as well as what type of information about use it provides, so that the results are not misunderstood (Reisfield, Webb, Bertholf, Sloan, & Wilson, 2007). For example, a patient taking codeine and acetaminophen as prescribed may test positive for both codeine and morphine. Also, the rates of false positive and false negative testing can be high with urine drug tests, and if the collection of specimens is not observed, it is possible for patients to submit urine samples that are not their own. Having confirmatory testing available, particularly if important treatment decisions are based on these results, is vital.

Feedback

Following the screening process, patients should be provided with feedback about the screening. Within the SBIRT framework, the following information is generally provided to patients: (a) objective information about the results of the screening, (b) recommended next steps, and (c) general guidelines about use of alcohol and drugs.

Results From Screening

The first step—screening—identifies the patient's risk level for substance-related problems. Patients who had negative screens are considered low risk and are not exceeding recommended guidelines for alcohol and are not using illicit drugs or using prescription medications for nonmedical reasons. Sharing this good news with the patient is an opportunity to highlight patients' strengths, encourage ongoing healthy habits, and perhaps prevent future risky or harmful substance use.

Patients who have positive screens for alcohol or drugs should be informed of their results and risk levels. They also should receive information about recommendations for how best to proceed based on their risk level (see the Interventions section of this chapter for further information on risk levels and recommended interventions). The feedback process also includes sharing information about general guidelines for use of alcohol and drugs. In general, this would be sharing the National Institute on Alcohol Abuse and Alcoholism (NIAAA) guidelines for daily and weekly alcohol consumption (see Chapter 1, this volume, for guidelines), as well as the guideline for no use of illicit drugs or using prescription medications for nonmedical reasons or in a way that is not prescribed. However, based on the setting or the patient's medical condition, the recommendations may change. For example, patients with certain medical conditions (e.g., liver disease), patients who are pregnant or may become pregnant, and patients who are taking medications that contraindicate alcohol use may be advised to abstain and provided with additional information about why any alcohol use is risky.

How to Share Feedback

Just as important as the feedback shared with the patient is how feedback is shared. Feedback should always be provided in a patient-centered manner. Consistent with the practices and principles of motivational interviewing (Miller & Rollnick, 2013), it is recommended that clinicians first ask a patient's permission to share feedback. Asking permission enhances collaboration, equalizes power in the therapeutic relationship, and increases willingness to hear feedback that may be difficult to hear. Feedback should be provided in user-friendly language, free of complex medical or mental health jargon. Finally, it is vitally important that feedback is shared in an empathic, nonjudgmental manner. Given the stigma and potential legal issues surrounding substance use, going to great lengths to demonstrate compassion and a desire to collaboratively help patients will reduce opportunities for creating discord in the therapeutic relationship.

Interventions

After sharing appropriate feedback with the patient, the next step is to help the patient receive the appropriate level of intervention. Patients who are abstinent or at low risk generally don't require any intervention outside of providing positive reinforcement and validation of their low-risk behavior. For those in the at-risk, high-risk, or dependent categories, different levels of intervention are required.

At-Risk Substance Use

Patients in the at-risk category generally are exceeding recommended alcohol guidelines and/or are using drugs at a level that may not yet be causing significant problems. These patients either do not meet criteria for a substance use disorder or, if they do, are in the mild category. Patients whose screening reveals that they are at risk of developing alcohol- or drug-related problems due to their current consumption patterns receive a brief motivational intervention. Research shows that about 16% of patients screened in a primary care setting will be exceeding recommended guidelines for alcohol or have illicit drug use within the past 30 days, and the vast majority of patients who have a positive screen will be in this category (Madras et al., 2009).

Brief motivational interventions are based on principles of motivational interviewing (Miller & Rollnick, 2013) and are designed to increase the internal motivation of the patient to reduce substance use to nonharmful levels. These strategies (Bien, Miller, & Tonigan, 1993) are commonly summarized as FRAMES (Feedback on individual risk level, patient Responsibility for change, Advice on need to change, using a Menu of choices, Empathy from the provider, and increasing Self-efficacy). Strategies to avoid when delivering a brief motivational intervention include anything that might be perceived as confrontational or noncollaborative such as lecturing, threatening, and giving advice or recommendations without first asking permission. In addition to the book written by Miller and Rollnick (2013), there are other books that provide quick tips and strategies for delivering brief motivational interventions in a variety of contexts (Rollnick, Miller, & Butler, 2007; Schumacher & Madson, 2015).

High-Risk Substance Use

Patients in the high-risk category are already experiencing alcohol- or drug-related problems and may meet criteria for a mild to moderate substance use disorder. The appropriate intervention for this group is a brief treatment, consisting of up to six to eight weekly sessions (Madras et al., 2009) that go beyond a brief motivational intervention to also include further assessment, education, problem solving, and developing coping strategies, problem-solving strategies, and a plan for addressing high-risk situations related to their use. In many instances, this level of care is not available within the medical setting where the screening occurred and requires a referral to a mental health or substance abuse treatment program. However, having the ability to provide this level of intervention within the medical setting is highly advantageous in that patients are already familiar with the clinic and may be more likely to follow-up appropriately if they can return to the same clinic for this service. This level of intervention is generally not provided by a medical provider. An allied health-care professional, such as a clinical health psychologist, is an ideal provider for this brief treatment.

As with all interventions, brief treatments should be evidence based (see Chapter 3 for a review).

The World Health Organization has created a guide for patients and providers for cutting down or stopping substances that is appropriate for patients at the high-risk level (Humeniuk, Henry-Edwards, Ali, Poznyak, & Monteiro, 2010b). This manual has been used by some sites when implementing SBIRT; it is easy to use and is free of charge. In their study of the SAMHSA SBIRT implementation, Madras et al. (2009) found that 3.2% of patients screened were in the high-risk category and were referred for a brief treatment episode.

Dependent Substance Use

For patients at the highest risk level—dependent—they are already experiencing significant problems related to substances and are likely to meet criteria for a moderate to severe substance use disorder. The recommendation is for these patients to be referred to a substance use specialty treatment program. This level of treatment could include a residential or inpatient treatment setting or an intensive outpatient treatment program. Generally, residential treatment programs are best suited for the most complex patients with medical or other psychiatric comorbidities requiring the structure of an around-the-clock treatment program and team. For patients with few or less complex medical comorbidities, an intensive outpatient treatment program, in which the patient can live at home or a location outside of the treatment facility, is likely to be adequate. The outcome research comparing residential treatment with intensive outpatient treatment shows equivalent outcomes across these treatment settings (Guydish, Werdegar, Sorensen, Clark, & Acampora, 1998). (See Chapter 3, this volume, for additional information on determining the appropriate level of care for patients.)

Referral to Treatment

Patients in the high-risk and dependent categories are likely to need referral to more specialized treatment, though some integrated care clinics may be able to provide appropriate services to those in the high-risk category. Being able to make a good referral to a treatment program is vital, and frustrations with providers are likely to develop when substance use problems are identified but viable treatment options are not available. Developing working relationships with mental health and substance use treatment programs in the catchment area greatly enhances a provider's ability to successfully place patients into care. In our experience, taking the time to proactively reach out to treatment programs and develop collaborative relationships is key to success. During a busy clinic, attempting to contact multiple treatment programs to which a patient could potentially be referred is challenging; having established relationships with substance use treatment programs can frequently make the referral process seamless and much less stressful. It is particularly important to identify treatment programs that use evidence-based interventions. Unfortunately, there are many substance abuse treatment programs that use interventions without empirical support or have treatment philosophies contraindicated for successful addiction treatment (Fletcher, 2013). The SAMHSA treatment locator (https://www.findtreatment.samhsa.gov/) or the NIAAA treatment locator (https://alcoholtreatment.niaaa.nih.gov/) are publicly available resources for assistance.

RESEARCH FINDINGS

Findings from the SAMHSA SBIRT initiative show excellent outcomes. In the first outcome review of findings, Madras et al. (2009) found that for those who used illicit drugs at baseline, rates of drug use at 6-month follow-up were statistically significantly lower by 67.7% and heavy alcohol use was lower by 38.6%, also statistically significant. A recent reanalysis of the original SBIRT cohort found that alcohol use was reduced by 35.6%, heavy drinking by 43.4%, and illicit drug use by 75.8% at the 6-month follow-up point (Aldridge, Linford, & Bray, 2017). Randomized controlled trials of brief interventions consistently support their efficacy for reducing risky or harmful drinking (Platt et al., 2016), and there is also evidence that these approaches are cost-effective (Barbosa, Cowell, Bray, & Aldridge, 2015) in emergency and outpatient settings. However, the evidence that these approaches result in seeking additional treatment for alcohol is less clear and may reflect problems with the availability of appropriate services following referral (Glass et al., 2015). The data from a large randomized controlled trial are less supportive of the benefits of screening and brief intervention for illicit drug use and prescription misuse in primary care, but far less research has been devoted to this application and additional research is necessary (Saitz et al., 2014).

TIPS FOR IMPLEMENTATION

Integrating SBIRT into a medical setting requires not only clinical knowledge and skills but also an understanding of implementation science. Lessons learned from medical settings where SBIRT has already been successfully implemented can be valuable for guiding future implementations. SBIRT was implemented to 10 diverse primary care clinics who offered the following guidelines for implementation (Hargraves et al., 2017):

- Have a practice champion who is respected by coworkers and works effectively across providers and is supported by leadership.

- Use all members of the interprofessional team, from front desk personnel to information technology staff to medical and psychosocial providers, as this can minimize the strain on physicians and other clinicians tasked with implementation.

- Create detailed expectations and materials for all team members and communicate these expectations clearly.

- Develop relationships with referral partners to better connect patients to treatment.

- Integrate SBIRT training into new employee orientation and maintain ongoing professional training.

- Understand clinic flow and create ways to streamline SBIRT into existing processes.

- When possible, use prescreening questions to avoid doing more in-depth screenings when they are not needed.

- Use the electronic health record to support SBIRT by creating reminder systems, flags for positive screens, and to assist with billing.

SUMMARY

SBIRT is a relatively quick, evidence-based approach to assessing, preventing, and providing initial intervention for harmful substance use in medical settings. With the help of several initiatives from SAMHSA, training in this approach is widely available and is typically geared toward providers who have limited baseline knowledge in harmful substance use. Although SBIRT represents just the first step for the vast majority of patients who have developed a substance use disorder, particularly if it is in the moderate to severe range, without this step patients may continue harmful substance use for years with the physical, mental, and social consequences of use mounting and sometimes multiplying as the years progress.

PART II

PSYCHOLOGICAL ASSESSMENT AND INTERVENTION FOR COMMON COMORBID PROBLEMS

5 ASSESSMENT AND TREATMENT OF DEPRESSION

Many psychologists have probably heard that depression is the leading cause of disability worldwide (Friedrich, 2017). Many psychologists may be less aware, however, that alcohol and drug-use disorders are also associated with significant disability in the United States (Hasin, Stinson, Ogburn, & Grant, 2007) or that alcohol has been identified as a major preventable risk factor for chronic disease and injury worldwide (Rehm et al., 2009). In this chapter, the complex and reciprocal relationship between substance use and depression will be reviewed. Key findings of several large-scale population studies are summarized, followed by an overview of assessment of co-occurring depression and substance use. Finally, evidence-based interventions for depression in individuals with substance use are reviewed with a clinical vignette to illustrate these treatment principles.

http://dx.doi.org/10.1037/0000160-006
Psychological Treatment of Medical Patients Struggling With Harmful Substance Use,
by J. A. Schumacher and D. C. Williams

RELATIONSHIP BETWEEN DEPRESSION AND HARMFUL SUBSTANCE USE

Depression and substance use commonly co-occur. Practitioners often wonder, "Does misusing substances lead to depression, or do patients use substances as a way of coping with depression?" The answer is yes. The relationship between depression and substance use is complex and can be reciprocal. Research shows that depression can increase the likelihood of developing a substance use disorder, and conversely substance use disorders can affect depressive disorders, including causing them directly, as in the case of substance induced depressive disorders. Several large-scale population studies and meta-analyses shed considerable light on this complex relationship.

Prevalence of Depression and Substance Induced Depression

As described in Chapter 2 of this volume, the first wave of the National Epidemiologic Survey on Alcohol and Related Conditions (NESARC) was a cross-sectional survey of the population in the United States, collecting data on substance use disorders, risk factors, and other psychiatric disorders. Analysis of these data (Grant et al., 2004) has helped to determine the prevalence of depressive disorders compared to substance-induced depressive disorders. Substance-induced depressive disorders are relatively uncommon, accounting for less than 2% of respondents who met criteria for a depressive disorder within the past 12 months, meaning that co-occurring depression commonly co-occurs above and beyond the influences of substance intoxication and withdrawal. The lifetime prevalence of major depressive disorder (without a substance use disorder) was 7.41%, while the lifetime prevalence of comorbid major depressive disorder and substance use disorder was 5.82% and the lifetime prevalence of substance-induced depressive disorder was only 0.26% and thus relatively uncommon in the general population (Blanco et al., 2012).

Co-Occurrence of Substance Use Disorders and Depression

Findings from NESARC also show that individuals with a substance use disorder are more likely to have a mood disorder than individuals without a substance use disorder, particularly those with drug abuse and alcohol or drug dependence (*DSM–IV* nomenclature [American Psychiatric Association, 2000; Grant et al., 2004]). Nearly 20% of respondents with any substance use disorder also experienced at least one independent mood disorder during the same 12-month period, with major depressive disorder being the most common. Conversely, individuals with mood disorders are more likely to also have a substance use disorder. For respondents with any mood disorder in the past year, about 20% had at least one substance use disorder. Rates of co-occurrence tend to be higher in treatment-seeking populations, with approximately 40% of individuals seeking treatment for an alcohol use disorder also meeting criteria for a current independent mood disorder. This finding was even higher among those with a current drug-use disorder, with about 60% meeting criteria for at least one independent mood disorder. Analysis of data from participants in the Sequenced Treatment Alternatives to Relieve Depression study (STAR*D), a large study of treatment-seeking patients with major depressive disorder, found that 29.4% also met self-reported criteria for a substance use disorder (Davis et al., 2006).

Longitudinal epidemiological research reveals that not only do depression and substance use disorders co-occur but that having depression is a major risk factor for developing substance misuse. The National Comorbidity Study was a population survey of psychiatric and substance use disorders in the United States completed at two time points about 10 years apart (Swendsen et al., 2010). In that study, having any baseline mood disorder increased a respondent's chances of transitioning from being a nonregular substance user to a regular substance user, of progressing from regular use to alcohol or drug abuse, or progressing from substance abuse to dependence. Self-medication of mood symptoms may account for some of this risk. An analysis of Wave 1 NESARC data found that almost one fourth of individuals with mood disorders report using alcohol or drugs to self-medicate symptoms (Bolton, Robinson, & Sareen, 2009). Moreover, longitudinal examination of data from Waves 1 and 2 reveals that individuals who reported self-medication motives for drug use were almost 8 times more likely to develop a severe drug use disorder 3 years later (Lazareck et al., 2012).

Implications of Co-Occurring Substance Use and Depression

There are also clear indications from epidemiological research that co-occurring mood and substance use can be associated with a complex and severe clinical picture. Additional analysis of the first wave of NESARC data (Blanco et al., 2012) reveals that having co-occurring depression and substance abuse is more strongly associated with having additional psychiatric diagnoses, sleep problems, feelings of worthlessness, suicidal ideation, and suicide attempts than having a major depressive disorder without a co-occurring substance use disorder. These co-occurring individuals were more likely to be male, divorced, or never married, were younger age at the onset of first depressive episode, and had more previous suicide attempts and greater functional impairment. Findings from a meta-analysis show that 60.5% of individuals with above-average depression show above-average levels of current alcohol use and impairment, compared with 39.5% of those with below-average depression. Moreover, higher levels of alcohol use and impairment were associated with higher levels of depression at follow-up (Conner, Pinquart, & Gamble, 2009).

RESEARCH ON TREATING CO-OCCURRING DEPRESSION AND SUBSTANCE USE

There is a complex and reciprocal relationship between depression and substance use. Here, we review this relationship, as well as the evidence-based practices for treating these co-occurring disorders.

Effects of Treating Depression on Substance Use

Although there is evidence that mood disorders and a desire to self-medicate them increase risk for developing substance use disorders, research on treating depression in individuals with co-occurring substance use disorders typically reveals modest impact on substance use. A review summarized the clinical findings of treating co-occurring depression and alcohol use as "conclusions drawn for patients with depression were that both tricyclics and SSRIs alleviated depression in most but not all cases, but they had little effect, direct or otherwise, on reducing drinking" and "antidepressants alone do not typically appear to affect drinking in depressed alcohol-dependent patients" (Pettinati, O'Brien, & Dundon, 2013, pp. 6–7). Another summary of the empirical evidence concluded that "antidepressants (with psychosocial treatment) alleviate depressive symptoms but have relatively little impact on reducing alcohol drinking in the majority of the studies reviewed of patients with co-occurring depression and alcohol dependence" (Pettinati, 2004, p. 790). Meta-analytic research showed that "the effect of treating depression on substance abuse outcome appears limited, and among such dually diagnosed patients, therapies directly targeting the addiction are also needed" (Nunes & Levin, 2004, p. 1894).

Effects of Treating Substance Use on Depression

Quite in contrast to the findings about the effectives of treatment of depression on substance use outcomes, there is growing evidence that improvements in substance use disorder symptoms lead to improvements in depression symptoms. In an early study of individuals attending inpatient treatment for alcohol use disorder, clinically significant levels of depression were present in 42% of patients at intake, but only 6% of patients at the fourth week of treatment. The largest reduction in symptoms occurred at the second week of treatment (S. A. Brown & Schuckit, 1988). Hasin et al. (1996) examined the 5-year outcomes of individuals with comorbid depression and alcohol use disorder and found that remission from alcohol use disorder strongly increased the likelihood of remission from depression and reduced the likelihood of having a return to depressive episode.

A study of treating co-occurring depression and substance use disorder in a primary care clinic demonstrated the importance of treating substance use disorder as quickly as possible (Chan, Huang, Bradley, & Unützer, 2014). In this study, helping patients enter substance use treatment resulted in a significantly greater likelihood of depression improvement than was observed for patients who declined treatment or those who were not treated. Timeliness of referral was also important as each week delay in initiating treatment resulted in decrease in the likelihood of depression improving.

EBP for Co-Occurring Depression and Substance Use Disorder

Evidence-based psychotherapies for co-occurring depression and substance use disorder are emerging. A systematic review found five randomized controlled trials using manualized treatments for co-occurring depression and alcohol misuse (Baker, Thornton, Hiles, Hides, & Lubman, 2012). The researchers concluded that "there is evidence that psychological interventions [motivational interviewing (MI)/cognitive behavior therapy (CBT)] are effective for treating co-occurring mood or anxiety disorders and alcohol misuse" (Baker et al., 2012, p. 228). Longer interventions were associated with greater improvements in mood and alcohol use outcomes, but brief interventions still demonstrated some efficacy. Brief supportive psychotherapy and interpersonal psychotherapy were not found to be effective.

A meta-analysis (Riper et al., 2014) found 12 studies examining the effectiveness of combined CBT and MI to treat clinical and subclinical alcohol use disorder and major depressive disorders. Results indicate that combined CBT/MI interventions are effective at treating co-occurring major depressive disorder and alcohol use disorders. Effect sizes were small but clinically and statistically significant. Notably, the outcome effects on alcohol reduction improved over time, with improvements in depressed mood occurring earlier than the improvements in alcohol use.

In perhaps the most rigorous study to date examining the efficacy of an intervention for co-occurring alcohol and depression (Baker et al., 2014), patients were assigned to an MI session or an MI session plus nine further sessions of CBT either focused on alcohol, depression, or both. Outcomes were measured up to 36 months after the intervention. The results provided the strongest support for the integrated depression/alcohol group and the alcohol-only focused groups as both produced better alcohol-related outcomes than the depression-only group. The integrated intervention resulted in faster short-term improvement in depression symptoms while the alcohol-only group had the best outcome for days of heavy drinking.

Combined treatment for substance use and depression relies on a set of core evidence-based skills, including motivational enhancement, symptom monitoring, activity scheduling, mindfulness skills, cognitive restructuring, planning for emergencies, problem solving, and relapse prevention. The Depression and Alcohol Integrated and Single-focused Interventions (DAISI) treatment manual (Kay-Lambkin, Baker, Hunt, Kavanagh, & Bucci, 2005) serves as a model. Motivational enhancement sessions are based on principles of MI (Miller & Rollnick, 2013). Here, skills such as open-ended questions and strategic reflections are used to reduce ambivalence and increase internal motivation to reduce alcohol use and engage in treatment.

Symptom monitoring is a common strategy in cognitive behavior treatments and uses homework templates to track symptoms between sessions to better understand when symptoms occur, such as worsening mood or urges to use, as well as ongoing substance use.

Activity scheduling is derived from behavioral activation for depression (Dimidjian, Barrera, Martell, Muñoz, & Lewinsohn, 2011) and consists of identifying and scheduling activities that are pleasant, consistent with the client's values, and give a sense of mastery. Instead of waiting until mood improves and desire to engage in activities returns, activity scheduling dictates that scheduled activities are performed regardless of mood symptoms to increase activation and allow natural reinforcement to improve mood.

Mindfulness skills focus on the ability to be aware of and observe your own thoughts, physical sensations, and emotions. These skills can be applied to both depression and substance use. Exercises are completed to develop the ability to observe experience and no longer use unhelpful responses, such as substance use, as ways of coping with unpleasant experiences.

Both depression and substance use disorders may be recurrent problems and susceptible to identifiable triggers. Predictable triggers for both depression and substance use are identified, including strategies for assertively addressing them with healthy coping strategies to avert potential high-risk crisis situations.

Problem solving focuses on proactively addressing problems, particularly those that are high-risk situations for substance use and depression. A six-step problem-solving methodology is taught to help clients systematically and strategically address problems to counteract the impulsive or avoidant strategies commonly practiced by clients.

Relapse prevention focuses on teaching the client self-care strategies for increasing resilience to relapse to depression and substance use. It also helps the client create a written plan identifying early warning signs of relapse, summarizes effective strategies for intervening quickly, high-risk situations that could predict relapse, and skills for maintaining gains.

ASSESSING DEPRESSION WITH SUBSTANCE USE

It is important to note that some symptoms of depression can be caused by intoxication or withdrawal from a substance. Many depression-related symptoms are outlined in the *Diagnostic and Statistical Manual of Mental Disorders* (American Psychiatric Association, 2013a) as part of intoxication or withdrawal symptoms. For example, as alcohol levels decrease during intoxication, it is common to see depressed mood and social withdrawal. Patients withdrawing from heavy and prolonged cannabis use often experience sleep difficulty, decreased appetite, restlessness, and depressed mood. Opioid withdrawal commonly involves dysphoric mood and insomnia. In chronic amphetamine use, intoxication can be accompanied by blunted affect, fatigue, sadness, or social withdrawal, and amphetamine withdrawal may include insomnia or psychomotor retardation. Depression and suicidal ideation may occur in frequent, high-dose amphetamine users during withdrawal. Even tobacco withdrawal can create symptoms of depressed mood, poor concentration, and insomnia.

In medical settings, blood alcohol levels and urine or blood drug screens can be helpful in assessing for substance use that may not be readily apparent from the patient's behavioral presentation or self-report. As further discussed in Chapter 4, this volume, it is important to understand the limitations of drug testing to ensure that interpretation of the results is correct. For example, some tests have high levels of false positive results or don't detect certain substances. Also, withdrawal symptoms may continue to be present after blood alcohol levels and drug screens no longer detect the substance.

For diagnostic purposes, it is important to distinguish between substance-induced and primary depressive disorders. According to the *DSM–5*, a disorder is substance induced if it is due to the direct effects of the substance based on a one-month period in which the substance would be expected to create a depressive effect (American Psychiatric Association, 2013a). Indicators that the disorder is not substance induced include the depressive disorder chronologically preceding the substance use, the depressive disorder lasting longer than 1 month beyond the expected effects, or other evidence that the depression is better explained outside the substance use based on history or other relevant data (Pettinati et al., 2013).

To effectively diagnosis comorbid depression with harmful substance use or substance use disorder, a thorough clinical interview focused on ascertaining the timing of the depressive episodes compared with the timing of the effects of substances should be conducted. Grant and colleagues (2004) outline the clinical distinctions to diagnose a depressive disorder as independent or nonsubstance induced; in the depressive episode, one of the four following conditions should apply: (a) there was no substance use in the past 12 months, (b) the depressive episode did not occur in the context of substance intoxication or withdrawal, (c) the depressive episode occurred before alcohol or drug intoxication or withdrawal, or (d) the depressive episode began after the effects of intoxication or withdrawal but persisted for more than 1 month after the substance effects occurred.

Ideally, validated measures for depression should be added to diagnostic interviewing when assessing for depression in a patient with substance use. There are a variety of self-administered measures with strong validity and reliability, such as the Patient Health Questionnaire—9 (PHQ–9; Kroenke, Spitzer, & Williams, 2001), Beck Depression Inventory—II (BDI–II; A. T. Beck, Steer, & Brown, 1996), and the Center for Epidemiologic Studies Depression Scale (CES-D; Radloff, 1977). Some of these are available without charge.

CLINICAL VIGNETTE

Mr. Jones is a 47-year-old man presenting to his primary care provider for his annual physical. Mr. Jones has gained 15 pounds since his last physical and reports feeling "sluggish." His sleep is restless and his energy is poor, which he attributes to his high-stress job as a sales manager at a successful car dealership, where he works long hours. Dr. Rodgers, his primary care provider, runs usual laboratory testing and finds that his patient's blood pressure is elevated and his liver enzyme and blood sugar levels are higher than in the past. When asked about his drinking, Mr. Jones acknowledges drinking "a bit more" than in the past and that his wife has been "nagging" at him about stopping for a few drinks on the way home from work.

Given Mr. Jones's worsening laboratory findings, weight gain, and stress, Dr. Rodgers is concerned and refers Mr. Jones to the behavioral health consultant for a brief assessment. He is given several self-administered instruments to complete, including the Patient Health Questionnaire—9 (PHQ–9; Kroenke et al., 2001), the Alcohol Use Disorder Identification Test (USAUDIT; Babor et al., 2016), and a Generalized Anxiety Disorder—7 questionnaire (GAD–7; Spitzer, Kroenke, Williams, & Löwe, 2006). The results of the self-administered assessments revealed a PHQ–9 score of 19 (moderately-severe depression), a GAD–7 score of 4 (normal), and an AUDIT score of 13 (high risk). A brief structured interview finds that Mr. Jones meets criteria for Major Depressive Disorder, Moderate severity, and Moderate Alcohol Use Disorder. The primary care provider and the behavioral health consultant meet with Mr. Jones, share the results of their assessment, and recommend CBT for alcohol and depression. The primary care provider also offers to prescribe an anticraving medication and/or an antidepressant medication to assist with treatment. Mr. Jones consents to initiate CBT and accepts the primary care doctor's medications, starting on 20 mg of fluoxetine and 333 mg of acamprosate, three times per day.

Early sessions of CBT focus on motivational enhancement. While Mr. Jones appreciates that his alcohol consumption quickly helps him feel less stressed and "unwind" after work, he also discloses that his father had a heart attack at a young age and he is concerned that his current drinking may be leading him in the same direction. He also is worried about his relationship with his wife, who is concerned about his drinking and "grumpy mood," as well as his ability to be effective at work. Mr. Jones agrees to a drinking holiday—a period of abstinence from alcohol to see what positive effect this could have on his health and depressive symptoms. This is done in consultation with his primary care provider to ensure safe weaning from alcohol.

Middle sessions of CBT focus on monitoring his mood, activity levels, and increasing his engagement in pleasant activities. Tracking his activity levels reveals that many of Mr. Jones's former hobbies, such as playing on a recreation league softball team, slowed and then stopped as his work became more stressful and as he stopped more frequently at the bar than the softball field. Mr. Jones identifies several activities to start scheduling, such as going for a walk or bike ride with his wife. Tracking also reveals that his urges to drink were highly correlated with his stress levels at work and depressed mood. Sessions focused on more proactively managing stress at work and replacing his drinking with other mood-enhancing activities.

Cognitive restructuring also is used to address his cognitions related to drinking and depression. For alcohol, it is revealed that he is prone to thinking of alcohol as the solution to his problems with thoughts like, "I better stop for a drink to help me unwind from work." For depression, he tends to catastrophize and jump to conclusions: "If we don't make our sales quota this month I'll be fired for sure." He is taught to evaluate the evidence for and against his beliefs (e.g., his recent performance evaluation was positive) and develop thoughts based on the available evidence (e.g., "My boss told me good job after our last meeting").

Late sessions focus on relapse prevention skills. High-risk situations for drinking, such as work-related stress worsening, are identified, as well as strategies for healthy coping. Over the course of treatment his depressive symptoms improve significantly, with his PHQ–9 score decreasing from moderately-severe to mild. While Mr. Jones still has a drink periodically, his drinking is within low-risk drinking guidelines and reserved for planned drinking experiences as opposed to coping with stress.

6 ASSESSMENT AND TREATMENT OF ANXIETY

The prevalence of anxiety and trauma-related disorders is elevated in individuals with harmful substance use and, conversely, individuals with anxiety and trauma-related disorders are at increased risk for harmful substance use. It is important for psychologists who work with either of these issues to be aware of these patterns of co-occurrence and how co-occurrence may affect assessment or treatment. In this chapter, we review information about the co-occurrence of these issues, provide an overview of how to assess anxiety and related disorders in individuals with harmful substance use, and present a continuum of evidence-based approaches to treatment of anxiety and related disorders for patients with harmful substance use. A clinical vignette is used to illustrate the topic in a cardiac care patient.

CO-OCCURRENCE OF ANXIETY AND HARMFUL SUBSTANCE USE

Epidemiological surveys consistently show that anxiety disorders and trauma-related disorders co-occur with substance use disorders at greater rates than would be expected by chance alone. Based on U.S. epidemiological data,

http://dx.doi.org/10.1037/0000160-007
Psychological Treatment of Medical Patients Struggling With Harmful Substance Use,
by J. A. Schumacher and D. C. Williams

individuals with any lifetime drug use disorder are 1.5 times more likely to report posttraumatic stress disorder (PTSD) and 1.3 times more likely to report an anxiety disorder (Grant et al., 2016). Moreover, almost half of people who report lifetime generalized anxiety disorder will also report a lifetime substance use disorder and will have higher rates of other psychiatric disorders (Alegría et al., 2010). Similar findings emerge for alcohol use disorders and anxiety disorders across multiple epidemiological surveys. In general, individuals with anxiety disorders are 2.1 to 3.3 times more likely to have an alcohol use disorder than those without anxiety disorders, and the association is stronger for more severe alcohol use disorders (Smith & Randall, 2012). With regard to PTSD, just under one fourth of the estimated 6.4% of U.S. adults who meet criteria for lifetime PTSD also meet criteria for severe alcohol use disorder (*DSM–IV* alcohol dependence; Blanco et al., 2012). These data suggest that it is important to assess for co-occurring anxiety and trauma-related disorders in individuals with substance use disorders, and also to assess for co-occurring substance use problems in individuals who have an anxiety or trauma-related disorder.

In considering the co-occurrence of anxiety and trauma-related disorders with harmful substance use, an important question is whether alcohol and drugs somehow contribute to the development of anxiety disorders or whether anxiety disorders contribute to the development of alcohol and drug problems. There is evidence that both of these models may be important to understanding why these problems co-occur and that there may be variability in the applicability of the models across specific disorders. There is also evidence that regardless of etiology, once the disorders co-occur they may become mutually maintaining (Smith & Randall, 2012). Stewart and Conrod (2008) labeled this the "vicious cycle of comorbidity" between anxiety and substance use disorders. The case illustration provided at the end of the chapter depicts this mutual maintenance.

Harmful Substance Use As a Cause of Anxiety

During active substance use or in the period after recent discontinuation of use, individuals may experience anxiety or trauma symptoms as a direct result of substance use and withdrawal. In the fifth edition of the *Diagnostic and Statistical Manual of Mental Disorders* (*DSM–5*; American Psychiatric Association, 2013a), anxiety is a symptom of withdrawal for alcohol, cannabis, tobacco, and sedatives, hypnotics, or anxiolytics, and can be a symptom of caffeine, cannabis, hallucinogen, or stimulant intoxication. There is also evidence that cocaine and hallucinogen use can precipitate anxiety states and panic (Norton, Norton, Cox, & Belik, 2008). Moreover, cannabis use has been associated with a risk for earlier onset of panic disorder and cannabis dependence has been associated with a greater risk of panic attacks (Zvolensky et al., 2006). In the case of alcohol use disorders, there is evidence from the first wave of the NESARC that harmful alcohol use tends to precede the onset of generalized anxiety disorder and panic disorder, but tends to follow the onset of specific and social phobia (Falk, Yi, & Hilton, 2008). Thus, for some individuals, harmful substance use may precede the development of anxiety, but the opposite temporal sequence may also occur.

Self-Medication

In our own work with co-occurring disorders, many clients and patients report that they began or escalated their use of drugs or alcohol to cope with negative feelings. In the case of trauma, it is not uncommon for someone to cite a specific traumatic event such as the death of a loved one as a precipitant of the most recent relapse. These anecdotal reports are echoed in findings from the research literature that using substances to self-medicate symptoms is associated with increased risk for harmful use. In longitudinal epidemiological surveys, adults who endorsed symptoms but did not meet criteria for panic disorder, social phobia, specific phobia, or generalized anxiety disorder and also reported using alcohol or drugs to self-medicate those symptoms were up to 5 times more likely to report a new onset substance use disorder three years later than adults who had symptoms but denied self-medication (Robinson, Sareen, Cox, & Bolton, 2011). In a survey of individuals who use marijuana for self-medication, anxiety was one of the most commonly reported conditions that respondents were attempting to medicate (Osborn et al., 2015). Consistent with those survey findings, there is evidence that social anxiety disorder in adolescence or young adulthood can precede use of marijuana, and that marijuana smoking is an attempt to cope (Buckner, Bonn-Miller, Zvolensky, & Schmidt, 2007; Buckner et al., 2008).

Several studies also suggest that self-medication also plays a role in drinking among those with trauma-related disorders. For example, in a sample of recently battered women, those who reported heavy alcohol use reported more severe trauma symptoms than abstainers or moderate drinkers, and this association was mediated by reports of drinking to cope (Kaysen et al., 2007). Similarly, individuals who develop PTSD following potentially traumatic life experiences are more likely to expect tension reduction or other positive benefits from drinking than individuals who have similar experiences but do not develop PTSD. Furthermore, these differences in expectations are associated with alcohol-related problems (e.g., Bedard-Gilligan, Kaysen, Desai, & Lee, 2011; Hruska & Delahanty, 2012; Peters, Khondkaryan, & Sullivan, 2012).

When working with patients who report using substances to self-medicate trauma or anxiety, it is important to educate patients about the data suggesting that drugs and alcohol may make trauma and anxiety worse overall. For example, although cannabis is being used to self-medicate anxiety, there is currently limited evidence that cannabidiol and nabilone (both non-psychoactive marijuana derivatives) improve social anxiety and PTSD, respectively, but there is no evidence that cannabis itself is therapeutic for anxiety and trauma, and there is moderate evidence that regular cannabis use increases risk for developing social anxiety disorder (National Academies of Sciences, Engineering, and Medicine, 2017). There is also evidence that substances may cause anxiety states or disorders (Norton et al., 2008; Zvolensky et al., 2006), and as described below, there is evidence that sustained cessation of substance use in those with substance use disorders leads to improvements in anxiety and trauma (S. A. Brown, Irwin, & Schuckit, 1991; Coffey, Schumacher, Brady, & Cotton, 2007).

Assessing Anxiety and Related Disorders in Individuals With Harmful Substance Use

Because anxiety can be a symptom of substance intoxication or withdrawal, assessing anxiety in individuals with harmful substance use can be a challenge. In the work of our research group examining individuals in treatment for severe alcohol or cocaine use disorders who also had a history of trauma, we found that trauma-related symptoms declined over the first 28 days in treatment, with the most change occurring during the first 2 weeks of abstinence (Coffey et al., 2007). Similar findings have been observed for anxiety during inpatient treatment for alcohol use disorder (S. A. Brown et al., 1991). This phenomenon may lead to overdiagnosis of anxiety or trauma-related disorders in individuals who are newly abstinent from a substance. This difficulty establishing an accurate co-occurring anxiety diagnosis may be especially problematic for substances with pronounced anxiety as part of the withdrawal syndrome such as alcohol and benzodiazepines (American Psychiatric Association, 2013a). Delaying evaluation for 2 weeks or more after cessation of substance use may facilitate more accurate assessment of co-occurring anxiety and trauma-related disorders. Another strategy for accurately establishing co-occurring symptoms may be to attend to nonoverlapping symptoms. For example, in the case of PTSD, whereas hyperarousal, avoidance, and negative alterations in mood or cognition might be a direct effect of substance use or withdrawal, reexperiencing is unlikely to be an effect of substance use or withdrawal (Read, Bollinger, & Sharkansky, 2003).

When assessing anxiety and trauma in individuals with co-occurring harmful substance use, it is also important to be aware that assessment of anxiety or trauma may briefly heighten symptoms by causing a patient to think about stimuli they normally avoid (Read et al., 2003). Read and colleagues (2003) encouraged clinicians to assess how anxiety and trauma symptoms relate to substance use (e.g., Are cravings for substance often triggered by anxiety or trauma symptoms?) and take steps to reduce risk for substance use if it is heightened by the assessment. For example, a clinician may assess less detail about trauma history or feared situations or integrate coping skills such as relaxation into the evaluation if there is reasonable concern that evaluation could trigger urges to use. These tips for assessing co-occurring anxiety and harmful substance use are summarized in Exhibit 6.1.

TREATMENT OF CO-OCCURRING HARMFUL SUBSTANCE USE AND ANXIETY

Many of the most-well-researched psychological treatments for trauma and anxiety disorders have been studied in individuals who are dually diagnosed with a substance use disorder. Although as outlined in Chapter 5, much of the research on treating co-occurring treatments for depression focuses on integrated treatment approaches, an important question in applying standard psychological treatments for trauma and anxiety to these individuals has been the appropriate sequencing of treatment. Should treatment be sequential, simultaneous, or integrated? These options are briefly described in Exhibit 6.2, and as Smith and Randall (2012) noted, there are pros and cons to each approach. For example, one advantage of sequential treatment

EXHIBIT 6.1. Tips for Assessing Anxiety and Trauma in Patients With Harmful Substance Use

- If possible, delay assessment until patient has approximately two weeks of nonuse.
- Be aware of overlapping symptoms such as hyperarousal or sleep disturbance, and look for nonoverlapping symptoms such as reexperiencing to support diagnostic impressions.
- Ask patients specifically about how substance use is influenced by anxiety or trauma.

EXHIBIT 6.2. Treatment Sequencing Options for Individuals With Co-Occurring Disorders

- **Sequential treatment** typically involves providing treatment for substance use disorder and then addressing the co-occurring anxiety or trauma-related disorder often at a different facility and after some delay.
- **Simultaneous treatment** refers to providing treatment for both the substance use disorder and the anxiety or trauma-related disorder at the same time, but not necessarily by the same provider or facility.
- **Integrated treatment** occurs when a single provider treats or at least monitors both the substance use disorder and the anxiety or trauma-related disorder simultaneously.

---

is that anxiety or trauma symptom reduction that occurs naturally as an individual has a greater number of days of nonuse of substance may eliminate the need for the second treatment (S. A. Brown et al., 1991; Coffey et al., 2007). On the other hand, if an individual's use of drugs or alcohol is triggered by anxiety or trauma symptoms, they may be more likely to resume use if they complete substance treatment without addressing the anxiety or trauma. Moreover, there is risk that some individuals who would have engaged in simultaneous or integrated treatment will drop out prior to or fail to return for anxiety or trauma treatment due to the extended treatment course necessitated by the sequential model. Simultaneous treatment addresses the mutual maintenance and extended treatment course concerns somewhat, but participating in two complete treatments simultaneously can be overwhelming for the patients, particularly if the approaches include between-session assignments. As is the case for depression, integrated treatment is often viewed as ideal for efficiently addressing both conditions as well as the mutual maintenance of the conditions, but not all patients are interested in addressing both problems and, as outlined in the introduction, few providers are equipped to address both problems. When treatment is not integrated, we recommended that the various care components be overseen and monitored by a single provider. For example, a patient in primary care who is identified as needing treatment for panic disorder and an alcohol use disorder might receive a prescription for an SSRI from the primary care provider, a referral to an in-house psychologist-led anxiety skills group, and a referral to brief substance use treatment at a nearby substance use treatment facility. The primary care provider would then monitor symptoms and progress in all treatments at follow-ups. Management of simultaneous care is illustrated in the clinical vignette in Chapter 8.

Exposure-Based Therapy

Exposure to feared or avoided stimuli is an active treatment ingredient in many evidence-based treatments across the spectrum of anxiety disorders and PTSD (Olatunji, Cisler, & Deacon, 2010). There is evidence that the optimal sequencing of exposure-based therapy for individuals who are also engaging in harmful substance use may differ depending on the specific diagnosis. Although we often hear concerns from both mental health and substance use treatment providers that offering exposure-based trauma treatment in a simultaneous or integrated fashion to individuals with co-occurring substance use disorders leads to a return to substance use, research suggests that this sequencing is optimal for many individuals. There are several studies investigating use of simultaneous or integrated exposure-based treatment for PTSD in individuals with co-occurring substance use disorder, including some in which we have been involved, and the most typical finding is that participants who receive exposure experience improvements in both posttraumatic stress and harmful substance use and do not have worse substance use outcomes than those in comparison conditions (Coffey et al., 2016; Foa et al., 2013; Mills et al., 2012). Although not specific to exposure-based treatments, there is some evidence that those who receive trauma treatment may be less likely to complete treatment than those who only complete substance use treatment (Roberts, Roberts, Jones, & Bisson, 2016).

There is also evidence that exposure-based treatments for panic disorder can be used in those with co-occurring substance use disorders without worsening substance outcomes, although it is unclear whether these treatments improve anxiety outcomes beyond substance use disorder treatment alone (Toneatto & Rector, 2008). The cautionary tale in the use of exposure for anxiety-related disorders comes from a randomized controlled trial of an exposure-based treatment for co-occurring social anxiety and alcohol use disorder. This study found that all participants had improvements in anxiety and some improvements in alcohol, but alcohol-related outcomes were worse at 3-month follow-up for the group that received exposure (Randall, Thomas, & Thevos, 2001). Although it is unclear why this occurred, it may be that participants who received the treatments were more likely to place themselves in social situations that triggered urges to drink than those in the other group. Overall, the research suggests that concurrent or integrated exposure-based treatment is likely to enhance outcomes for individuals with co-occurring posttraumatic stress disorder without increasing risk for substance relapse. The research on anxiety disorders is less clear and suggests that a sequential approach might be more prudent in some cases until more research evidence emerges. A sequential approach helps ensure that substance use symptoms have been addressed and stabilized before anxiety symptoms are addressed. Alternatively, a longer period of continuing care for substance use disorder might be recommended for those with co-occurring anxiety, especially social anxiety.

Cognitive Therapy

Cognitive therapy focuses on directly modifying maladaptive cognitions that maintain anxiety or trauma symptoms. Cognitive processing therapy is an evidence-based intervention for PTSD that incorporates cognitive therapy and written trauma exposure accounts and has typically shown equivalent PTSD symptom reduction outcomes to exposure-based treatment (Resick, Nishith, Weaver, Astin, & Feuer, 2002). Cognitive processing therapy been used in veterans with and without current or past alcohol use disorders, and a large medical record review study found no difference in treatment completion and significant reductions in depression and PTSD for both groups (Kaysen et al., 2014). For patients who are reluctant to discuss their trauma directly, a version of cognitive processing therapy that excludes the written trauma account has demonstrated efficacy in patients without co-occurring substance use disorders (Resick et al., 2008) and may be efficacious for patients with co-occurring harmful alcohol use (McCarthy & Petrakis, 2011). Although there are limited studies examining the effects of cognitive therapy apart from exposure for anxiety, among studies testing this effect, there is evidence that effects of cognitive therapy and exposure are equivalent for panic disorder and may be superior for social phobia (Ougrin, 2011). Importantly, the treatment outcome literature on cognitive therapy for trauma and anxiety specifically in those with co-occurring substance use disorders is limited at this time, and future research is needed to guide decisions about their use, especially in patients with active substance use disorder.

Mindfulness and Relaxation

Mindfulness-based interventions and relaxation training are commonly used in the treatment of anxiety and trauma-related disorders, but their benefits for those with co-occurring substance use disorders are less clear. In those without dual diagnoses, mindfulness-based interventions for anxiety show promising evidence and appear to have effects similar to those of cognitive behavior therapy and superior to approaches such as supportive therapy or relaxation (Hofmann, Sawyer, Witt, & Oh, 2010; Khoury et al., 2013). These approaches integrate mindfulness practices that help a patient cultivate a mental state in which they are nonjudgmentally aware of the present moment. This mental state is thought to counter the future focus that characterizes anxiety and can also facilitate a greater willingness to experience thoughts and feelings rather than avoiding them. There is promising but inconclusive evidence for these approaches in the treatment of PTSD (King et al., 2013). Mindfulness meditation has also been examined as a treatment for substance use disorder, but there is insufficient data to conclude whether substance use outcomes are improved by these interventions (Zgierska et al., 2009).

Relaxation training includes a broad variety of cognitive or behavioral strategies designed to help patients develop a relaxation response to counteract a stress response. Relaxation training is typically found to be an efficacious treatment for various forms of anxiety, but typically has inferior outcomes to full cognitive behavioral therapies when directly compared (Manzoni, Pagnini, Castelnuovo, & Molinari, 2008; Olatunji et al., 2010). Although their efficacy for those experiencing harmful substance use as well as anxiety or PTSD is unclear, various relaxation strategies such as breathing retraining, progressive muscle relaxation, or visualization might reasonably be offered as stand-alone treatment to provide a patient with tools for managing anxiety or trauma symptoms for those who do not desire or cannot access other treatments. They may also be offered as a coping skill for patients who are or will be receiving sequential rather than integrated treatment for harmful substance use and anxiety or trauma-stressor related disorders.

Pharmacotherapy

A comprehensive review of pharmacotherapy for co-occurring harmful substance use and anxiety is beyond the scope of this chapter. However, we feel it is important to devote some attention to prescription benzodiazepines such as alprazolam and clonazepam, which are Schedule IV controlled substances under the Controlled Substances Act (Drug Enforcement Agency, 2017). Although these medications have demonstrated safety and efficacy for the short-term treatment of anxiety, they are generally considered inappropriate for individuals who have co-occurring harmful alcohol or drug use out of concerns that they may be misused (Marshall, 2008). One important exception is their use in the acute treatment of alcohol withdrawal following brief, specified, tapering schedules. Among patients who are prescribed benzodiazepines for anxiety, ongoing assessment can be important to ensure that appropriate use does not transition to harmful use. In a community sample of 67 adults who were prescribed anxiolytic or sedative drugs for anxiety or sleep, over 50% of participants reported misusing their prescription on at least one occasion with the most common forms of misuse being exceeding recommended dose for therapeutic (42%) or nontherapeutic (21%) reasons and taking their prescription medication with another substance such as alcohol, cannabis, or stimulants (40%). Additionally, more than 50% reported diverting their prescription on at least one occasion (McLarnon, Monaghan, Stewart, & Barrett, 2011). There is limited research on individuals with co-occurring harmful substance use and anxiety to guide selection of pharmacotherapy, but existing evidence generally supports the use of SSRIs or buspirone with co-occurring alcohol use disorder and anxiety (Marshall, 2008).

CLINICAL VIGNETTE

Peter Collins is a 55-year-old man who has been followed in cardiology for 5 years subsequent to a heart attack. He has come in recently complaining of increased chest pain. During triage he was asked about his use of alcohol and drugs, and he reported having one to two drinks each evening and smoking marijuana three to four times per week for the past year to help him reduce his stress. Given the positive screen for harmful substance use, he is referred to a clinical health psychologist for further evaluation. When he meets with the psychologist, he is asked more about the stress he is experiencing. He reports that stress related to paying for his children's college and losses in the stock market have made it hard for him to relax for the last few years. He further reports that he has begun having periods of acute anxiety during which he experiences panic-like symptoms, such as racing heart and shortness of breath. When asked about the pros and cons of marijuana use, he reports that on the one hand he likes the way it makes him feel and on the other hand he worries that it might actually be causing some of his cardiac symptoms, that it is contributing to marital problems because his wife, who is "straight-laced," does not approve of his marijuana use, and he always has in the back of his mind that he could lose his job if he gets drug tested at work.

Smoked marijuana is known to increase risk for chest pain and acute cardiac events in individuals diagnosed with heart disease. Heavy use may also induce panic-like symptoms. There is also evidence that although he uses marijuana to help him cope with stress and worry, marijuana use itself is contributing to Mr. Collins's stress and worry. Thus, an important first step in addressing his anxiety and worry is getting him to reduce, or preferably stop, smoking marijuana. To this end, the psychologist teaches Mr. Collins a variety of relaxation tools, such as breathing retraining and progressive muscle relaxation, as a means for better managing his stress and reducing his panic-like symptoms. As Mr. Collins learns to better apply relaxation techniques, he begins to be more aware of his worries—especially about his finances. The psychologist helps Mr. Collins articulate his worries (e.g., "I'm going to go broke paying for my kids' college") and evaluate how well they fit with the objective evidence. The psychologist and Mr. Collins note that Mr. Collins was prone to fortune telling—predicting negative outcomes without evidence to support them—and needs to work on thinking more evenly about the future based on the evidence available. As Mr. Collins progresses with these skills, the psychologist introduces some practical strategies for limiting access to marijuana and engaging in alternative strategies when he has the urge to use. Mr. Collins no longer keeps marijuana at home and better communicates with his family about his financial concerns. As a result, he is able to reduce his marijuana use significantly and feels less compelled to smoke in order to manage his stress. His episodes of angina, heart palpitations, and trouble breathing show notable improvements as well. He also reports feeling better about himself and his relationship with his wife, and he reports that he likes going to work without having to worry about whether he will get selected for a drug screen.

7

ASSESSMENT AND TREATMENT OF SLEEP DYSREGULATION

Findings from epidemiological research suggest that many Americans have some problem with sleep. For example, results of one survey place the prevalence of both feeling unrested during the day and not getting enough sleep at night at just over one fourth of the population (Ram, Seirawan, Kumar, & Clark, 2010). However, a much smaller percentage of the population experiences sufficient symptoms to meet full diagnostic criteria for a sleep disorder. Three common sleep disorders—insomnia, restless leg syndrome, and sleep apnea—are experienced by 1.2%, 0.4%, and 4.2% of the population, respectively (Ram et al., 2010). Although fairly common in the U.S. population, sleep dysregulation is almost ubiquitous in individuals who engage in harmful substance use, particularly those with substance use disorders. The most commonly reported problem among those with substance use disorders is insomnia (i.e., difficulty initiating or maintaining sleep or sleep that is nonrefreshing; Roehrs & Roth, 2015; Substance Abuse and Mental Health Services Association, 2014).

http://dx.doi.org/10.1037/0000160-008
Psychological Treatment of Medical Patients Struggling With Harmful Substance Use,
by J. A. Schumacher and D. C. Williams

We begin this chapter with a brief overview of sleep and sleep disorders for readers who may be less familiar with this area. After this general overview, we review the literature on the comorbidity of sleep dysregulation and harmful substance use. We then provide practical guidance on addressing co-occurring sleep problems and harmful substance use including formal and informal strategies for assessing sleep dysregulation, unique concerns related to pharmacotherapy for sleep in individuals with harmful substance use, and sleep hygiene techniques and other evidence-based behavioral strategies to improve sleep. At the conclusion of the chapter a clinical vignette is used to illustrate this topic in a primary care patient.

SLEEP AND SLEEP DISORDERS

During normal sleep, an individual cycles through three stages of non-rapid eye movement sleep (N1, N2, & N3) as well as rapid eye movement (REM) sleep. N1 (formerly Stage 1) sleep is a light stage of sleep experienced as the person is drifting off to sleep. Individuals are easily aroused during N1. N2 (formerly Stage 2) usually follows N1 and represents a deeper sleep. N3 (formerly Stages 3 and 4) is the deepest stage of sleep, characterized by slower brain waves and during which it is typically difficult to rouse the individual, and they are likely to be confused if awakened. REM sleep is the stage of sleep associated with dreaming, and brain waves are much more similar to waking than during other phases of sleep. A complete sleep cycle takes an average of 90 to 110 minutes, and over the course of the night Stage 3 sleep gets shorter and REM sleep gets longer. These sleep stages and cycles are sometimes referred to as sleep architecture, and each stage of sleep appears to be important for optimal daytime functioning (Institute of Medicine, 2006; National Sleep Foundation, 2019; Perlis, Jungquist, Smith, & Posner, 2005; Roehrs & Roth, 2001).

The fifth edition of the *Diagnostic and Statistical Manual of Mental Disorders (DSM–5)* includes 10 disorders or disorder groups in the Sleep–Wake Disorders section (American Psychiatric Association, 2013a). Although the specific symptoms of each disorder or disorder group vary, individuals seeking treatment for sleep–wake disorder often present with a similar list of list concerns: dissatisfaction about quality, quantity, or timing of sleep and daytime distress and impairment. (Note: *DSM–5* classification is intended for use by general clinicians rather than sleep specialists. Sleep specialists often use the *International Classification of Sleep Disorders, Third Edition*; American Academy of Sleep Medicine, 2014). Three common physician-diagnosed sleep disorders are (a) breathing-related sleep disorders (e.g., obstructive sleep apnea), which are characterized by breathing disturbances in sleep that result in daytime sleepiness or fatigue; (b) insomnia disorder, which is characterized by difficulty initiating or maintaining sleep resulting in daytime distress or impairment; and (c) restless legs syndrome, which is characterized by an urge to move the legs particularly at night or during periods of rest, which results in distress or impairment (American Psychiatric Association, 2013a; Ram et al., 2010).

SLEEP DISTURBANCE AND SUBSTANCE USE

Epidemiological studies demonstrate associations between insomnia-type sleep disturbances and alcohol and substance use and use disorders (Roane & Taylor, 2008). As detailed in this section, this relationship seems to be both complex and bidirectional.

Sleep Problems As Risk Factors for Substance Use

There is evidence that sleep problems often precede or predict the onset of harmful substance use. For example, childhood sleep problems predict alcohol and drug outcomes in adolescence and young adulthood for some youth (Wong, Brower, Nigg, & Zucker, 2010). Among individuals in recovery from alcohol use disorder who also experience sleep problems, over half may have developed the sleep problem prior to the onset of the alcohol use disorder or used substances to sleep (Currie, Clark, Rimac, & Malhotra, 2003). Among individuals currently in alcohol use disorder treatment, more than 60% may experience insomnia, and of those, more than half may specifically use alcohol to facilitate sleep (Brower, Aldrich, Robinson, Zucker, & Greden, 2001). Poor sleep is also a key predictor of relapse for individuals with alcohol use disorder (Brower, 2015; Brower et al., 2001) and can interfere with cannabis quit attempts (Babson, Boden, Harris, Stickle, & Bonn-Miller, 2013). Moreover, sleep dysregulation has often been shown to persist following treatment and discontinuation of drugs or alcohol after prolonged use can cause REM sleep rebound or rebound insomnia (Roehrs & Roth, 2015; Substance Abuse and Mental Health Services Administration, 2014).

Patients with sleep-related problems may find substance use more reinforcing, which may facilitate escalation of substance use. For example, for individuals with insomnia or hyperarousal (a common daytime correlate of insomnia), cannabis, sedative-hypnotics, and alcohol use may be negatively reinforced by relief from this unpleasant state. Similarly, for individuals who experience daytime sleepiness or fatigue, stimulants, caffeine, or nicotine may be more reinforcing. In these cases, continued use, difficulty reducing use, and resumption of use after periods of abstinence may represent self-medication (Roehrs & Roth, 2015).

Substance Use As a Risk Factor for Sleep Problems

During active use or withdrawal, drugs and alcohol can impair sleep directly causing problems with falling asleep, maintaining sleep, and modifying sleep architecture (Brower et al., 2001; Roehrs & Roth, 2015). In *DSM–5*, all of the identified withdrawal syndromes for substances (i.e., alcohol, caffeine, cannabis, opioids, sedative/hypnotic/anxiolytic, stimulant, tobacco) include sleep disturbance or daytime drowsiness or fatigue as a potential symptom (American Psychiatric Association, 2013a). Alcohol deserves a bit of special attention in this section as many people report having a "nightcap" before bed to help them sleep. While there is evidence that low doses of alcohol may be beneficial for sleep, higher doses disrupt sleep during the second half of the night. Moreover, there is evidence that tolerance to alcohol's sedative effects may develop quickly (Roehrs & Roth, 2001). *DSM–5* also includes a diagnostic category specifically for substance/medication-induced sleep disorders (American Psychiatric Association, 2013a). This diagnosis applies to prominent and severe disturbance in sleep (i.e., insomnia, daytime sleepiness, and/or parasomnia) with an onset that can be linked directly to substance intoxication or withdrawal. Importantly, these sleep disorders can be diagnosed whether or not the individual also has a use disorder related to the substance that induced the sleep disturbance.

Given the direct impact of substances on sleep, it is not surprising that many patients with substance use disorders report dysregulated sleep. In one small study, 96% of individuals seeking treatment for substance use disorders (primarily alcohol and/or opioids) had some level of sleep dysregulation as assessed with a structured measure, with over half reporting moderate to severe impairment, over half reporting symptoms of sleep apnea, and one third reporting symptoms of restless leg syndrome (Mahfoud, Talih, Streem, & Budur, 2009).

ASSESSING SLEEP DISTURBANCE

Assessing sleep disturbance requires a framework for conceptualizing what represents a sleep disturbance versus normal variation in sleep. In many ways, this framework parallels the one applied to alcohol and other substance use. For example, in thinking about whether or not someone who consumes alcohol has an alcohol problem and, if so, whether and what types of treatment they might need, it is important to consider how much alcohol the individual consumes. However, simply knowing that an individual consumes amounts of alcohol that exceed recommended guidelines or even consumes amounts of alcohol that lead to intoxication is an insufficient basis for diagnosis or treatment recommendations. Similarly, although there are general guidelines for amounts of sleep that are likely to be healthy for most adults, sleep needs are actually highly variable (Banks & Dinges, 2007; Edinger & Carney, 2008). Even knowing that an individual currently gets much less sleep than they previously did is insufficient information to determine that sleep is a problem. If the amount of sleep an individual is getting leaves them feeling rested and restored, does not cause any daytime impairment such as mood lability or difficulty concentrating, and is not associated with distress (e.g., complaints about sleep), regardless of what the quantity is, sleep is unlikely to populate our problem list for that patient.

When assessing sleep disturbance, it is important to be aware of and assess for lifestyle and environmental factors that influence sleep. The lifestyle and environmental factors that seem to promote optimal sleep are often referred to as good sleep hygiene. Although further information on sleep hygiene is provided in the section of this chapter on treatment, it is generally recommended that individuals maintain a consistent sleep schedule, in a cool, dark, quiet environment, that has been set aside for sleep, and do not engage in behaviors known to disrupt sleep (Mastin, Bryson, & Corwyn, 2006). To the extent that a patient engages in behaviors known to disrupt sleep, such as drinking caffeinated beverages just before bedtime or has an environment not conducive to sleep, such as a noisy bed partner, sleep dysregulation may be readily explained and remedied.

A number of psychometrically validated tools are available for assessing sleep disturbances. Some of these measures may be freely reproduced with permission for certain purposes. We commonly use the following three:

- Pittsburgh Sleep Quality Index (PSQI). The PSQI is 19-item self-rated assessment tool that includes items assessing sleep quality and disturbances over the prior month (Buysse, Reynolds, Monk, Berman, & Kupfer, 1989). Seven subscale scores can be calculated: (a) perceived sleep quality, (b) sleep onset latency, (c) sleep duration, (d) sleep efficiency, (e) sleep disturbances and perceived causes, (f) use of sleep medication, and (g) daytime impairment. Available online (https://www.sleep.pitt.edu/instruments/).

- Insomnia Severity Index (ISI). The seven-item ISI assesses perceived severity of sleep difficulties over the past 2 weeks including problems with sleep onset and maintenance as well as distress and impairment (Bastien,

Vallières, & Morin, 2001; Morin, 1993). Scoring and interpretation guidelines allow for categorization of patients in four categories: (a) no clinically significant insomnia, (b) subthreshold insomnia, (c) clinical insomnia (moderate severity), and (d) clinical insomnia (severe). Available online (https://eprovide.mapi-trust.org/instruments/insomnia-severity-index).

- Sleep Diary. A sleep diary is often used to gather specific information about sleep and monitor progress in patients who are receiving behavioral interventions for sleep (e.g., Edinger & Carney, 2008; Morin & Espie, 2004; Perlis et al., 2005). Patients complete the sleep diary daily and typically include information such as when they go to bed; how long it takes them to fall asleep; when they awaken; when they get out of bed; how often and for how long they awaken during the middle of the night; any medications, alcohol, or caffeine consumed at or near bedtime; and how they feel in the morning. This information allows the clinician to calculate important information about sleep such as sleep onset latency, wake after sleep onset, total sleep time, and sleep efficiency. Diaries may also include other information depending on what is pertinent to a particular patient such as naps, prebedtime behavior, exercise, cognitions about sleep, and estimated sleep quality. Printable sleep diaries are available online from websites such as the National Sleep Foundation (sleepfoundation.org).

In the absence of formal tools, a few key questions can offer significant clinical insights into the nature of a particular individual's sleep difficulties:

- *Do you have trouble falling asleep?* Estimates of more than 30 minutes to fall asleep on 3 or more nights per week is generally considered excessive sleep onset latency (Lichstein, Durrence, Taylor, Bush, & Riedel, 2003). Sleep onset difficulties may be common in individuals with problematic alcohol use (Currie et al., 2003).

- *Do you wake during the night?* Although normal sleep is characterized by brief arousals throughout the night between sleep cycles, these typically are not recalled by the individual. Sleep loss of 30 minutes or more due to wake after sleep onset on 3 or more nights per week is generally considered excessive (Lichstein et al., 2003).

- *Do you awaken before the desired time?* Awakening too early in the morning and being unable to fall back to sleep is sometimes called *late insomnia.*

- *What are your sleeping habits like?* Specific questions may include: When do you go to bed? When do you arise? How long after you awaken do you stay in bed before arising? This enables a calculation of sleep efficiency, which is defined as the ratio of total sleep time to time in bed. In general, a sleep efficiency of 90% (e.g., 90% or more of the time in bed is spent asleep) is targeted as optimal because it limits opportunities for the bed and bedroom to become associated with arousal (Perlis et al., 2005).

- *Do you nap?* Although it is important to be mindful of cross-cultural differences, napping is often an indication that nighttime sleep is insufficient. If an individual seems to be getting a sufficient quantity of sleep at night and still requires daytime naps, it is important to ask follow-up questions about potential signs of breathing-related sleep disorder (e.g., snoring), periodic limb movement disorder, or restless leg syndrome.

- *How long has this been going on?* Although sleep may be a target for intervention in the absence of a diagnosable sleep disorder, to diagnose persistent insomnia, symptoms must have persisted at least 3 days per week for 3 months.

In addressing sleep and substance use, it is important for clinicians to assess specifically how substance use may affect sleep as well as how sleep may affect substance use. It is also important to be aware of the potential for other disorders to complicate the presentation. Sleep disturbance can be a symptom of many disorders and has been identified as a potential transdiagnostic mechanism that may account for high rates of comorbidity among disorders (Harvey, Murray, Chandler, & Soehner, 2011). In research on co-occurring alcohol and trauma symptoms in individuals in residential substance use disorders treatment with which we have been directly involved, insomnia was uniquely associated with the severity of trauma, alcohol, depression, and anxiety symptom severity even after controlling for emotion dysregulation (Fairholme et al., 2013). In patients who engage in harmful substance use, it is important to ask how sleep problems may differ during periods of active use or withdrawal relative to periods of nonuse, whether they currently use or started using substances to cope with sleep difficulties, whether they believe their substance use affects their sleep, and which substances they use and how they use them.

INTERVENTIONS

In this section, we describe intervention strategies for co-occurring sleep disturbance and substance use. As mental health professionals vary in their familiarity with cognitive behavioral therapy for insomnia, we provide detail about some of the elements commonly included in this intervention.

Abuse Liability in Sleep Medications

Lichstein and colleagues (2013) noted that although expert panels have cautioned against the use of hypnotics for long-term management of insomnia since the late 1970s and early 1980s, hypnotic use has continued to increase. In general, nonmedication treatments for sleep are preferred for individuals with harmful substance use, because many of the prescription medications approved by the U.S. Food and Drug Administration for the treatment of insomnia have the potential for misuse. Prescription benzodiazepine sedative-hypnotics such as triazolam and nonbenzodiazepine sedative-hypnotics such as zaleplon, escopiclone, and zolpidem are Schedule IV controlled substances under the Controlled Substances Act (Drug Enforcement Agency, 2017; Substance Abuse and Mental Health Services Administration, 2014). Even when used as prescribed, long-term sedative hypnotic use creates risk for physical and psychological dependence on the medications. Given that hypnotics are the most widely advertised and widely used sleep medications, patients seeking treatment may be misperceived by providers as "drug-seeking" if they have harmful substance use histories (Roehrs & Roth, 2015). Although the body of research supporting their efficacy for insomnia is underdeveloped, a number of unscheduled medications, including several antidepressants with sedating effects, have been prescribed off-label (for purposes other than the FDA's approved use) to individuals with harmful substance use and may represent an important alternative (Substance Abuse and Mental Health Services Administration, 2014).

Nonmedication Approaches to Sleep Dysregulation

Cognitive behavior therapy for insomnia is an evidence-based treatment that is often recommended as first-line treatment for insomnia (Morin et al., 1999; Trauer, Qian, Doyle, Rajaratnam, & Cunnington, 2015). Some of the common approaches include stimulus control, sleep restriction, relaxation, cognitive therapy, and sleep hygiene education. With the exception of sleep hygiene, these approaches can be used alone in the treatment of chronic insomnia (Morgenthaler et al., 2006) but are often used in combination in multicomponent cognitive behavioral therapy protocols (e.g., Edinger & Carney, 2008; Morin & Espie, 2004; Perlis et al., 2005). As with the literature on use of medications to treat sleep disturbance in individuals with harmful substance use, the literature on behavioral interventions is similarly limited. However, there have been multiple trials of cognitive behavioral therapy for insomnia in individuals with alcohol use disorder with promising effects, and there is at least one promising study for these interventions in individuals with other substance use disorders (Arnedt, Conroy, Armitage,

& Brower, 2011; Currie, Clark, Hodgins, & El-Guebaly, 2004; Roehrs & Roth, 2015).

The behavioral model of insomnia, which underlies the intervention strategies presented later, posits the interplay of predisposing, precipitating, and perpetuating factors in the development and maintenance of insomnia over time (Perlis et al., 2005; Spielman, Caruso, & Glovinsky, 1987). Predisposing factors are anything that might make a particular individual more likely to develop insomnia such as an inherently weaker sleep system, a tendency to worry or ruminate, or a sleep schedule that is mismatched to biological rhythms. Precipitating factors are acute events that interact with predisposition to cause acute insomnia such as a substance withdrawal syndrome, psychological stressors, or abrupt changes in sleep schedule such as the sleeping in that can accompany harmful substance use. Insomnia sparked by precipitating factors would be transient, the model posits, were it not for perpetuating factors. Perpetuating factors are maladaptive coping strategies adopted to manage acute insomnia. These strategies include things like spending more time in bed, engaging in nonsleep behaviors in the bedroom like reading, watching television, or worrying, or drinking alcohol at bedtime. Cognitive behavior therapy addresses the perpetuating factors that maintain chronic insomnia. A few common strategies are outlined next, but interested readers are encouraged to review one of many available treatment guides (e.g., Edinger & Carney, 2008; Morin & Espie, 2004; Perlis et al., 2005).

Sleep Hygiene

Sleep hygiene involves providing patients with psychoeducation about factors that promote and inhibit sleep and encouraging them to modify lifestyle and environmental factors to maximize the likelihood of sleep. Lifestyle factors include things such as limiting caffeine, alcohol, and nicotine use before bedtime; avoiding an overly full or empty stomach at bedtime; and exercising during the day but not so late in the day that it causes arousal at bedtime. Environmental factors include making sure the bedroom is cool, quiet, and dark and the bed is comfortable. Sometimes achieving an environment conducive to sleep requires introduction of items such as ear plugs or sound generators to manage outside noises or noisy bed partners, eye masks or dark curtains to block excess light, a fan to cool the room, and new sheets, pillows, or mattress to create a comfortable sleeping space.

Stimulus Control

Stimulus control involves helping the patient reduce associations that may have developed between the bed and bedtime and wakefulness. In this approach the patient is instructed to go to bed only when tired and to use their bed only for sleeping and sexual activity. Activities such as reading, watching television, or worrying in bed are prohibited. If the patient cannot fall asleep within 15 to 20 minutes or awakens for more than 15 to 20 minutes during the night, they are instructed to get up, go to another room, and engage in a quiet, nonstimulating activity, such as reading or listening to music. When they feel sleepy again, they are to return to the bed. Exiting the bedroom should occur any time the patient is awake more than 15 to 20 minutes during the night. It is important to note that stimulus control, particularly when combined with instructions to maintain a consistent bedtime and arising time, can result in increased sleep deprivation for a brief period. Therefore, it may be contraindicated for patients with bipolar disorder, seizure disorder, sleep apnea, or other conditions that may be worsened by sleep restriction. With patients who have co-occurring substance use, it is important to discuss whether sleep deprivation and accompanying daytime sleepiness may heighten urges to use substances.

Relaxation

To promote sleep, it is useful for patients to allow themselves an opportunity to wind down before bedtime with a presleep routine. In fact, in some research in which we were involved, a four-session intervention focused primarily on helping patients create a relaxing presleep routine had measurable impacts on sleep and daytime functioning (Wickwire, Schumacher, & Clarke, 2009). A typical presleep routine involves identifying a time that is an hour or more before bedtime during which the patient stops work, planning, and other activities and shifts to relaxing activities such as watching television or reading. The presleep period ends with a particular sequence of activities such as changing into pajamas, washing face, and brushing teeth that immediately precede going to bed and help signal bedtime. Typical relaxation exercises such as progressive muscle relaxation or breathing exercises may be incorporated into the presleep routine or used one their own to promote relaxation and sleepiness (Perlis et al., 2005). Patients may also find these strategies useful for managing urges to use substances or coping with negative affect triggers for use.

CLINICAL VIGNETTE

Michael Storm is a 60-year-old retired man who recently moved and established primary care with a new physician who was closer to his new home. As the physician took his history and asked if there was anything she needed to know, Mr. Storm reported that he has trouble sleeping and wondered whether a medication might help. His physician heard that cognitive behavioral therapy is often considered a first-line treatment for insomnia and referred Mr. Storm to a clinical health psychologist for evaluation and possible treatment of insomnia.

During his evaluation by the psychologist, Mr. Storm reveals that he developed insomnia approximately 15 years ago when his plant underwent significant layoffs. He would often lie awake for hours at night unable to turn his mind off. The insomnia has persisted despite the fact that his job situation was secured after about six months, and he has not experienced any significant worries or stressors since that time. When asked if he has found anything helpful, he reported finding that a drink or two before bed seems to help, but for quite some time he has noticed that he tosses and turns in the middle of the night and wakes up feeling nonrefreshed. As the psychologist further assesses Mr. Storm's drinking he finds that Mr. Strom's "drink or two" is actually four to eight standard drinks per night. He drinks whiskey from a standard 16-ounce glass and pours about 2 inches of whiskey into the glass before adding ice. About half the time he will go to bed after one drink, but half the time he still does not feel sleepy and will prepare a second drink. He denies any alcohol-related problems and his score on the Alcohol Use Disorders Identification Test, Adapted for Use in the United States places him in the "at-risk" category (Babor et al., 2016).

Mr. Storm's insomnia fits patterns that are common for chronic insomnia that co-occurs with harmful alcohol use. The insomnia began acutely with a stressful life event—layoffs at his plant 15 years ago—but has transitioned to chronic insomnia so that now, even though his stresses are reduced and he lives in a quiet peaceful setting, his sleep problems persist. Given that sleep problems are risk factors for harmful alcohol use, it is not surprising that he used alcohol to try to self-medicate this problem. Although alcohol seemed to help his sleep initially and continues to facilitate sleep onset, he now notices middle-of-the-night disruptions in sleep that are often common with higher doses of alcohol. Given the quantity Mr. Storm now drinks (up to eight standard drinks per occasion) and the duration of his drinking, it is likely that he is highly tolerant to the effects of alcohol.

Mr. Storm does not need specialty care for alcohol, so the psychologist delivers a brief intervention for harmful alcohol use to create a plan for cutting down on his drinking. Given the potential for withdrawal from alcohol with abrupt decreases or cessation, this plan for cutting down is created in collaboration with his referring physician. Because he is using alcohol primarily to sleep, Mr. Storm's plan for cutting down on alcohol includes scheduling additional meetings with the psychologist to learn cognitive behavioral strategies to improve his sleep. The psychologist first helps Mr. Storm begin monitoring his sleep using a sleep diary. The psychologist then teaches Mr. Storm progressive muscle relaxation and encourages him to use this practice to help him relax before bedtime and if he awakens during the night. Mr. Storm also begins taking morning walks to get exercise and early exposure to sunlight, both of which may enhance his ability to sleep at night. Within a few visits, Mr. Storm has cut his alcohol consumption to one to two standard drinks per night and reports that his sleep seems "much better" and that he feels "ready to face the day when he awakens." These reports are consistent with his sleep diary entries.

8 PSYCHOLOGICAL TREATMENT OF THE FAMILY

The quality of family relationships can influence harmful substance use, and harmful substance use can in turn affect family members (Copello, Velleman, & Templeton, 2005). It is important for clinicians who are working with patients who are engaging in harmful substance use to be aware of these reciprocal relationships and available options to address the needs of family members as well as patients. This chapter focuses on the needs of families in whom substance use occurs, the role of family and friend support in helping individuals to make changes in harmful substance use, and evidence-based treatment options for harmful alcohol and drug use that explicitly incorporate family. The chapter presents information on three of the most widely known interventions that focus specifically on the family members of those who engage in harmful alcohol and drug use: Al-Anon, Johnson Institute Interventions, and Community Reinforcement and Family Training. A clinical vignette is used to illustrate this topic in a women's health patient.

http://dx.doi.org/10.1037/0000160-009
Psychological Treatment of Medical Patients Struggling With Harmful Substance Use, by J. A. Schumacher and D. C. Williams

HARMFUL SUBSTANCE USE AND THE FAMILY

Health psychologists who work with individuals who do not engage in harmful substance use will likely still have to address harmful substance use in their practice. This is because families are often significantly affected by loved ones' substance use. In fact, it has been argued that although it is not counted as such, addiction in the family significantly affects the global burden of poor health through the stress and pain it causes (Orford, Velleman, Natera, Templeton, & Copello, 2013). Harmful alcohol and drug use may be associated with disruptions to family rituals, roles, routines, social life, finances, and communication (Copello et al., 2005). In addition to these disruptions, families of those who engage in harmful alcohol and drug use often report having to deal with things like intimate partner violence, child abuse, driving under the influence, and disappearing for days on end. A common story we hear in our own clinical practice is the parent of an adult child with a substance use disorder who has had money or medications stolen by their child, worries about their child's whereabouts, has had to call the police to seek protection from their child, or has even lost their child to overdose or substance-related illness or injuries.

When working with patients in whom harmful substance use has been identified, it is important to determine whether other family members are likely to support reductions in substance use. In some cases, patients may have limited family support due to family estrangements or discord, geographic disbursements, small family size, or other factors. In other cases, patients may live with family members who also engage in harmful substance use. In these cases, interventions specifically designed to help those with substance problems develop social networks that support changes in substance use may improve treatment outcomes, particularly for older adults (Beattie & Longabaugh, 1999; Litt, Kadden, Kabela-Cormier, & Petry, 2009; Schumacher, Stafford, Beadnell, & Crisafulli, 2018; Wasserman, Stewart, & Delucchi, 2001).

In our work delivering brief interventions for harmful substance use, we often help patients consider who could support them in making changes in their harmful substance use, whether they could reestablish contact with friends or family members who would support changes if none currently exist in the social network, and how they can reduce contact with those who might make it difficult for them to change their harmful substance use. Given decades of research, including our own, demonstrating an association between harmful substance use and both perpetration against and victimization by an intimate partner (Capaldi, Knoble, Shortt, & Kim, 2012; Schumacher, Feldbau-Kohn, Slep, & Heyman, 2001), safety assessment is an important part of working with both individuals who engage in harmful substance use and their family members. Safety assessment in best accomplished in a 1:1 interaction and usually includes straightforward questions about whether the individual has been harmed or fears harm from a partner or family member. Many individuals, women in particular, who need treatment for harmful substance may also need advocacy, safety planning, and other services for intimate partner aggression (Schumacher & Holt, 2012). These services will often require outreach to local domestic violence agencies. Pregnant and postpartum women with substance use disorders may be particularly likely to experience intimate partner aggression, and available evidence including some of our own work with this population suggests that they often have few treatment options (Dworkin et al., 2017; S. L. Martin, Beaumont, & Kupper, 2003). Conversely, the partners and families of individuals engaging in harmful substance use may need safety planning, advocacy, or other services to address violence that have experienced. Substance use treatment facilities are often best equipped to provide that help. In addition to determining the need for violence-specific resources, assessment of partner aggression perpetration and victimization can help clinicians decide whether the potential benefits of family-based treatment outweigh the risks. The Agency for Healthcare Research and Quality provides links to several partner violence screening tools on their website that can be used to facilitate safety assessment (https://www.ahrq.gov/professionals/prevention-chronic-care/healthier-pregnancy/preventive/partnerviolence.html).

COMMON TREATMENT OPTIONS FOR FAMILY MEMBERS

In this section, we describe three treatment options for family members: (a) Al-Anon Family Groups, which are widely available mutual self-help groups that actively discourage trying to change another's drinking or drug use and instead focus on the stresses of living with someone who has a substance use problem; (b) Johnson Institute Intervention, which trains the social network of an individual engaging in harmful substance to stage a confrontation to reduce denial and get them engaged in treatment; and (c) Community Reinforcement and Family Training, which teaches family members skills that help them influence their loved one's substance use and engage them in treatment.

Al-Anon Family Groups

Timko, Young, and Moos (2012) provided an in-depth overview of the features, characteristics, and research support for Al-Anon Family Groups. They noted that as Alcoholics Anonymous was beginning in the mid to late 1930s as a treatment option for individuals with alcohol problems (see Chapter 3 of this book), groups of concerned significant others were gathering informally for mutual support while their loved one attended an AA meeting. Al-Anon Family Groups, often referred to simply as Al-Anon, was formally founded in 1951. Al-Anon Family Groups is a mutual-help organization for relatives and friends of people who are engaged in harmful alcohol or drug use. Nar-Anon was formally incorporated in 1971 to provide a place for mutual support for individuals struggling with another's drug use. Alateen is an affiliate of Al-Anon for young people. The goal of these groups is to help and support concerned significant others who are affected by another person's drinking or drug use through opportunities to share experiences.

Al-Anon is widely available but may not be the right option for all patients or patient families struggling with another's harmful alcohol and drug use. Al-Anon often frames family members as codependent, meaning they are preoccupied with their loved one's behavior in the same way the loved one is preoccupied with alcohol or drugs (Timko et al., 2012). Family members are actively discouraged from trying to change another's drinking or drug use and instead to detach from that individual and focus on coping with the stresses of living with someone who has a substance use problem. As is typical in AA, Al-Anon members are encouraged to attend face-to-face meetings that may begin with a reading of the 12 steps and one or more of the 12 traditions and then focus on a particular topic and close with the Serenity Prayer. In addition to attending meetings, members are encouraged work the 12 steps, obtain a sponsor, develop spiritual practices, and become familiar with Al-Anon literature.

Although surveys of Al-Anon members support its positive benefits, there are few robust studies of its benefits. It is likely that it enhances coping both with a loved one's drinking and other stressors and may reduce psychological symptoms and negative emotion (O'Farrell & Clements, 2012; O'Farrell & Fals-Stewart, 2003; Timko, Laudet, & Moos, 2016; Timko et al., 2012). Not surprising, given that it is not the focus, Al-Anon does not appear to help the loved ones of concerned others enter treatment (Miller, Meyers, & Tonigan, 1999). We have worked with patients who have described Al-Anon as helpful as well as patients who do not desire to detach from their loved one or even feel that it is inconsistent with their core values to do so and prefer approaches that provide skills for directly addressing their loved ones' substance use such as the Community Reinforcement and Family Training approach described later.

Johnson Institute Interventions

Johnson Institute Interventions have been highly popularized by reality television shows depicting dramatic confrontation of individuals engaging in harmful alcohol and drug use. As reviewed by Copello and colleagues (2005), in this approach the social network of an individual who is engaging in harmful alcohol use is trained to stage a confrontation to reduce the individual's denial of the problems stemming from their alcohol use and engage them in treatment. However, a 2003 review of marital and family interventions for alcohol found only two studies documenting the success of this approach and a 2012 review identified no additional studies (O'Farrell & Clements, 2012; O'Farrell & Fals-Stewart, 2003). These reviews noted that the two available studies showed that these interventions only resulted in successful treatment engagement of a loved one 25% to 30% of the time because most families did not follow through with the confrontation. Thus, the authors concluded that there are insufficient data to recommend this approach to families who are concerned about a loved one's alcohol or drug use. There is also evidence that relapse rates may be high and treatment retention low following these confrontations (Copello et al., 2005).

Community Reinforcement and Family Training

Community Reinforcement and Family Training (CRAFT) is based on the idea that concerned significant others can affect a loved one's alcohol and drug use as well as their decision to enter treatment. The intervention largely focuses on teaching family members skills to accomplish these changes (Meyers, Miller, Hill, & Tonigan, 1998). Family members are taught skills for maintaining safety and preventing dangerous situations, how to reinforce nonusing behaviors to try to extinguish harmful substance use, social and problem-solving skills, planning activities and practicing strategies that interfere with the loved one's drug use, preparing to initiate treatment when a loved one seems ready, and supporting the loved one in treatment. The approach also includes elements to help family members improve their own quality of life. Reviews of outcome literature suggest that CRAFT results in family members getting a loved one to engage in treatment for harmful substance use about 68% of the time (O'Farrell & Clements, 2012; O'Farrell & Fals-Stewart, 2003). In a head-to-head comparison of Al-Anon, Johnson Institute Intervention, and CRAFT for the loved ones of individuals engaged in harmful alcohol use, the treatments resulted in a loved one getting treatment 13%, 30%, and 64% of the time, respectively (Miller, Meyers, & Tonigan, 1999). Although the treatment is designed to improve coping and reduce stress in family members, and could reasonably be expected to produce those benefits, the research on this approach does not tend to focus on this outcome. In studies that examine whether CRAFT enhances the functioning of family members, there is evidence that it leads to self-reported improvements in outcomes such as depression, anger, and family cohesion/conflict, but it is not superior to Al-Anon or Johnson Style Interventions in that regard (Roozen, de Waart, & van der Kroft, 2010).

Because CRAFT is not as widely available as other options, providers might encourage families to read the self-help book written by developers R. J. Meyers and B. L. Wolfe, *Get Your Loved One Sober: Alternatives to Nagging, Pleading, and Threatening* (2003).

CLINICAL VIGNETTE

Tanya Minton is a 23-year-old woman. She presents during the second trimester of her pregnancy for prenatal care at a women's specialty clinic. Her initial urine toxicology is positive for cocaine. When questioned about the toxicology results, she does not deny using cocaine and says she wants to do right by her baby, but she needs help. Further assessment reveals that Ms. Minton has been using drugs and alcohol since the age of 14 and cocaine specifically for approximately five years. She also reveals that the baby's father is a drug dealer and that when he is angry he sometimes hits her in the stomach. During the exam bruises on both arms from being grabbed roughly are noted.

Given the lack of coordination among substance use disorder, domestic violence, and prenatal care services in most communities, as well as the mandatory report to child protective services that is required in this state, this represents a challenging case. As a result, a psychologist is consulted. As the psychologist assesses the needs of Ms. Minton, maintaining safety while also addressing cocaine use are primary concerns. Given her cocaine use and her late access of prenatal care, her pregnancy is considered high risk and she will need more frequent prenatal care and monitoring to ensure her health and the health of her unborn child. She also is likely to need significant support as she works with the child protective system, but it will also be important to ensure she is aware that the psychologist is a mandated reporter. Based on a Posttraumatic Stress Disorder Checklist for *DSM–5* score of 53 (Blevins, Weathers, Davis, Witte, & Domino, 2015), Ms. Minton is experiencing significant trauma-related problems as well and would likely benefit from trauma treatment or at least a trauma-informed program.

When asked about social support, Ms. Minton reports that her mom does not talk to her anymore because she has "given up on her." She becomes teary and explains that she would like to go home, but she does not think her mom will take her back. Social work is not available to coordinate referrals or care in this setting, so the psychologist contacts the local domestic violence agency to see if a placement at a shelter may be possible for the duration of her pregnancy. Unfortunately, the local program does not have a linkage to substance use treatment and also does not provide shelter to women with active substance use disorders due to safety concerns. They are, however, willing to help Ms. Minton obtain a restraining order against the baby's father and develop a safety plan. They also have a counselor on staff that can provide trauma treatment. The psychologist next contacts a residential substance treatment facility in a community approximately 100 miles away that has a specialty substance treatment program for pregnant women. While this would be an optimal placement, the program does not currently have any beds available and does not anticipate an opening for 2 to 3 months. At this point, with gentle encouragement, Ms. Minton agrees to call her mother from the psychologist's office. The psychologist overhears a teary and intense phone call that results in Ms. Minton's mother agreeing that she can live with her at least until the baby is born but only if she gets treatment. The psychologist is able to get Ms. Minton a placement in a local day treatment program for substance use. Ms. Minton and the psychologist continue to meet monthly when Ms. Minton has prenatal appointments. These appointments focus on monitoring symptoms, managing stress, and applying problem-solving to any challenges Ms. Minton encounters as she tries to keep up with all the services she is receiving. Sometimes her mother attends these appointments to talk about the expectations she has for Ms. Minton and ways she can ensure her behavior is supporting Ms. Minton's continued abstinence rather than drug use, using a book recommended by the psychologist to support those goals. With these simultaneous treatments and services, Ms. Minton is able to maintain abstinence from cocaine throughout her pregnancy, has a reduction in trauma symptoms, and maintains a relationship with her mother that provides safe housing and support for managing the stresses of pregnancy and new motherhood.

9 RELAPSE PREVENTION AND CONTINUING CARE

Although often treated like acute illnesses, substance use disorders, much like diabetes, hypertension, and asthma, may be chronic, relapsing medical conditions that may require long-term care strategies (McLellan, Lewis, O'Brien, & Kleber, 2000). Following a treatment episode for substance use disorder is a particularly high-risk time for relapse. Developing interventions to avert or minimize returns to substance use after an acute treatment episode are important to allow maintenance of treatment gains. This chapter outlines traditional and widely available approaches to continuing care interventions and reviews the research literature on evidence-based interventions. Finally, a vignette demonstrates how these treatments could be applied to a patient in a cancer clinic.

TRADITIONAL TREATMENT MODEL

Historically, the traditional model of addiction treatment—the Minnesota Model—consisted of attending a 28-day inpatient or residential multidisciplinary treatment program, where the programming would be based

http://dx.doi.org/10.1037/0000160-010
Psychological Treatment of Medical Patients Struggling With Harmful Substance Use,
by J. A. Schumacher and D. C. Williams

on the 12-step model. This treatment would be followed by a transition to community 12-step meetings (Anderson, McGovern, & DuPont, 1999). This approach was progressive in that it conceptualized addiction as a treatable disorder and provided a treatment paradigm; however, it was limited in that it was rigidly focused on the 12 steps and a one-size-fits-all approach to treatment (McKay, 2009). Individuals needing treatment who did not agree with the 12 steps or desired more flexible treatment options were not well served by this model. While the Minnesota Model has evolved in terms of providing more treatment options (e.g., outpatient programs), the philosophical foundation of 12 steps has remained.

COMMON CONTINUING CARE MODELS

Mutual-Help Groups

As a result of the Minnesota Model, the most common form of continuing care is community mutual-help groups. Alcoholics Anonymous (AA) is the most common form of mutual help in North America and is widely available across the world (Humphreys, 2004). AA consists of networks of meetings, promoting a set of principles—the 12 steps—that serve as a roadmap for recovery from alcohol. Important AA principles include admitting powerlessness over alcohol; believing in and turning to a higher power for help, who can remove unhelpful character traits; recognizing and admitting previous mistakes and then trying to make amends for them, and actively maintaining a relationship with a higher power and using spirituality as a way to help others who need the 12 steps. A variety of accepted slogans capture essential AA principles, such as "turn it over," which encourages acceptance of things that can't be changed and encouragement to allow a higher power to guide you; "fake it till you make it," suggesting that following the AA process will lead to good outcomes and following it, even on faith, will be beneficial; and "one day at time," encouragement to make the focus on the most important thing today, not drinking.

Sponsors are laypeople, generally experienced in their own recovery, who serve as coaches to more inexperienced members to help them through the 12 steps and to be available to draw on their experience for the benefit of the member. There are rituals to begin and end meetings, such as common prayers (e.g., the Serenity Prayer), readings, or accepted sayings (e.g., "Keep coming back, it works if you work it right"). Some meetings feature speakers who tell their own story of recovery through the principles of AA. Other meetings allow members or other attendees to share their experiences informally with each other. Meetings generally have a member who presides over the group, providing it structure and guidance. There are approved reading materials for AA, including the *Big Book* and *Twelve-Steps and Twelve Traditions* (Alcoholics Anonymous, 1952, 2001). These books share the story, experiences, and philosophies of Bill W., a stockbroker, and Dr. Bob S., a physician, who founded AA in 1935. While there are commonalities across meetings, there is also wide variability in terms of accepted practices, expectations, and behavior in groups.

Other 12-step organizations have been created as offshoots to address other addiction-related behaviors, such as Narcotics Anonymous, Gamblers Anonymous, and Sexaholics Anonymous. There also has been a development of supportive groups for family members, based on the same principles, such as Al-Anon and Alateen (described in greater detail in Chapter 8, this volume). Twelve-step meetings don't charge membership fees, but they accept donations to fund meeting spaces, available literature, and other expenses. Anonymity is a principle of treatment in 12-step groups: "What is said here, stays here."

While the vast majority of self-help groups are based on the 12 steps, there are alternative groups with different philosophical foundations, such as Self-Management and Recovery Training (SMART Recovery). SMART Recovery is a program based on principles of rational emotive behavioral therapy. It focuses on increasing motivation to abstain from substances, changing unhelpful beliefs that lead to substance use, better learning to manage emotions that lead to substance use, and addressing problems and creating a lifestyle that supports recovery (http://www.smartrecovery.org/about). Meetings are available in person as well as online and, unlike 12-step groups, are led by trained facilitators. They also have resources for family members and loved ones of participants with online groups and message boards as well as referral to evidence-based resources for family members, including the Community Reinforcement Approach and Family Training (CRAFT) program (described in greater detail in Chapter 8). A variety of handbooks and materials are available to facilitators and participants to assist with their recovery process.

Counselor-Led Groups

Probably the most common form of continuing care, outside of community-based 12-step meetings, is 12-step-based groups associated with a treatment facility. Clients, following the completion of a primary treatment program, return on a regular basis—usually weekly or biweekly—for group therapy.

Similar to community 12-step meetings, these groups are focused on the 12 steps as the foundation for recovery. However, these groups are typically led by a counselor or therapist rather than a layperson. Unfortunately, research is lacking on this approach to continuing care. Research does show that over 50% of patients drop out of this continuing care by 3 months (McKay et al., 1999).

Research on Mutual Help

Unfortunately, empirical support for mutual-help groups is limited. Findings from the existing literature indicate that those who attend self-help programs and participate in related activities have better outcomes than those who don't participate in self-help activities (Kissin, McLeod, & McKay, 2003; Moos & Moos, 2007). A recent meta-analysis of dually diagnosed patients attending AA found that ongoing AA attendance was positively associated with abstinence up to 12 months after completing a treatment program (Tonigan, Pearson, Magill, & Hagler, 2018). A recent review of the SMART Recovery research literature (A. K. Beck et al., 2017) suggests positive effects based on a limited amount of research and the need for further, high-quality research to reach conclusions on outcome efficacy. Although the research on self-help groups is limited, given their broad availability (particularly 12-step groups), promising evidence for their benefits, and no clear evidence of iatrogenic or harmful effects, these may represent an important aftercare option for many patients.

Individual Psychotherapy

Project MATCH included the largest randomized controlled trial of manualized individual treatment as an aftercare approach for alcohol use disorders. This multisite study randomized patients, following an episode of intensive treatment (either residential or intensive outpatient treatment), to one of three conditions: twelve-step facilitation, cognitive behavioral therapy, or motivational enhancement therapy. Results demonstrate that these three approaches were equally effective (Project Match Research Group, 1997), with nearly 30% of participants abstinent from alcohol 3 years later and those who did report drinking showing a reduction of about 150% as measured in days abstinent (Project Match Research Group, 1998). Although these have not been subjected to the same rigorous evaluation as aftercare approaches for drug use disorders, they are considered evidence-based approaches for treatment of various drug use disorders (National Institute on Drug Abuse, 2018b). An advantage of these treatments is that, as part of federal research funding, each of these treatment manuals is publicly available. Each of these approaches is briefly reviewed.

Twelve-Step Facilitation

Unlike "working the 12-steps," in which a therapist helps guide a client sequentially through the 12 steps, Twelve-Step Facilitation (TSF) treatment is focused on helping patients better understand the 12 steps, including the jargon and key concepts, as well as problem-solving strategies for attending meetings, obtaining a sponsor, and other core ideas of the 12 steps (Nowinski et al., 1999). The TSF protocol consists of both "core" topics, which are covered with all patients, and optional topics that can be chosen based on the individual needs of the patient. The core topics include introducing the treatment program, reviewing the first three steps and their accompanying principles (acceptance and surrender), and the idea of "getting active" by proactively attending and participating in 12-step meetings and obtaining a sponsor.

Elective sessions focus on identifying substance-related problems across generations of families, stopping "enabling" behaviors that facilitate use by the client, changing routines and habits related to use, managing emotions connected with using, accepting responsibility for actions while not being overwhelmed by guilt, and developing a healthy sober lifestyle with good nutrition, hobbies, and exercise. The manual has two optional "conjoint" sessions for clients in relationships. For partners without a substance use problem, they are educated about resources available to them (e.g., Al-Anon), the principles of the 12 steps, how to avoid enabling the client's substance use, and finally allowing the client to experience the negative consequences of their substance use and not feeling guilt about not protecting the client from these problems. Importantly, each session also includes a review of the client's progress since last session, including the meetings they are attending, their sober days since last session, their urges to drink, any slips in their recovery, follow-up on assigned readings, progress on obtaining and using a sponsor, and reaching out to other members of the 12 steps for support and help.

Cognitive Behavior Therapy

The cognitive behavior therapy manual consists of both core and elective sessions (Kadden et al., 2003). There are more sessions available than expected to be provided, allowing for treatment to be individualized and tailored to the unique needs of the individual. It also includes two elective sessions for couples and family involvement.

There are eight core sessions, with an emphasis on identifying triggers to use, developing appropriate strategies for managing cravings, improved problem solving, assertive communication skills, coping with a return to use, and how small decisions can lead to use. Elective sessions focus on additional skills related to managing the connection between emotions and substance use (e.g., anger management, depression) as well as skills that help to improve the client's functioning beyond addiction (e.g., job-seeking skills).

Motivational Enhancement Therapy

Motivational enhancement therapy (MET) is shorter than the other individual treatment options and consists of only four sessions (Miller, Zweben, DiClemente, & Rychtarik, 1999). The first session of MET consists of obtaining objective information from the patient (and a significant other if possible) about their alcohol use and related problems, and providing them with an individualized feedback form that compares their use and problems with others and objective metrics, such as the peak blood alcohol level, risk factors, serum blood laboratory results (e.g., liver enzymes), negative consequences, and neuropsychology functioning.

The remaining sessions are focused on building the client's motivation to maintain changes made during their treatment program, as well as any additional changes they would like to make. Unlike other treatment approaches where the primary modality is educational or skill building, in MET the focus is on eliciting and strengthening the client's motivations for changing. A nonjudgmental attitude is essential and is combined with open questions, empathic listening, affirmations for strengths and efforts, responding with understanding to any sense of defensiveness. A change plan is developed for patients based on the patient's motivations and strategies for obtaining those goals. Information and recommendations are only made either by request from the patient or after asking the patient's permission.

Emerging Approaches

Stepped-Care Approach

While the previous models for aftercare attendance focus on providing the same treatment protocols to all patients, stepped-care approaches focus on providing the lowest level of care required and titrating amounts of care based on client need. One stepped-care approach to continuing care, developed by McKay and colleagues (2010), starts by providing telephone-based contacts between a therapist and the client, weekly at first (for the initial 8 weeks), twice monthly (next 10 months) and then titrating down to once per month (last 6 months). When clients' face significant risk factors for relapse, or do relapse, they are provided with several in-person sessions to enhance motivation, a more intensive relapse prevention protocol, or the option to return to a primary treatment program.

A randomized controlled trial of this intervention (McKay et al., 2010) revealed favorable outcomes for alcohol use disorder, with fewer days of alcohol use or days of heavy alcohol use in a month, up to 18 months after starting the continuing care intervention. However, the 24-month outcomes were not better than treatment as usual except for women and those with lower levels of readiness to change.

Contracts, Prompts, and Reinforcement

Research by Lash and colleagues (2007) combines several behavioral components into a comprehensive continuing care intervention designed to keep clients engaged in continuing care to improve outcomes. It combines the use of contracts, prompts (reminders), and low-cost reinforcers for participation (e.g., sobriety token, participation certificate). Within this protocol, clients who are completing primary addiction treatment sign a contract, identifying how much continuing care they would like to participate in. Then, during the continuing care, they receive reminders through the mail about attending their continuing care meetings. Finally, they creatively use reinforcers for meeting targeted goals, such as providing a certificate or sobriety token in group to a participant, and encouraging social reinforcement from other group participants to provide positive feedback about the participant's progress. While the evidence on the effectiveness of this approach is mixed (Lash et al., 2013), clients in this approach were more likely to complete at least 3 months of continuing care, remained in treatment longer, and were more likely to be abstinent from substances 12 months after starting the continuing care intervention.

Overall Research Findings on Continuing Care

Attempting to predict which patients will relapse, or which characteristics of patients will likely lead to relapse, has led to inconsistent results. A systematic analysis revealed that severity of alcohol dependence, severity of psychopathology, alcohol-related self-efficacy, motivation, and treatment goal were the most consistent predictors of outcome for patients with alcohol use disorder (Adamson, Sellman, & Frampton, 2009).

Research on continuing care interventions shows that overall, these interventions produce statistically significant results but with relatively small effect sizes. A recent meta-analysis (Blodgett, Maisel, Fuh, Wilbourne, & Finney, 2014) identified 33 controlled trials that included continuing care interventions and found that "gauged across a wide variety of treatments and at different time points, continuing care has a positive, although limited, impact on substance use outcomes" (p. 94) both at the end of the continuing care intervention and at follow-up. The study did not find any association between outcome and either length or intensity of the continuing care intervention. The limited number of controlled trials on continuing care interventions limited the ability of the meta-analysis to detect differences or determine which continuing care components may be the most potent. Further research on continuing care interventions is needed.

CLINICAL VIGNETTE

John Parker was seen in the cancer clinic after a series of medical appointments to determine the cause of his recent physical complaints. Mr. Parker originally presented to a community substance treatment program with a long history of alcohol use disorder. Providers initially attributed his physical complaints to the effects of alcohol or withdrawal symptoms. However, his symptoms persisted after completing detoxification and several weeks of intensive outpatient treatment.

Dr. Freeman, the health psychologist working with the cancer clinic, was consulted. Dr. Freeman worked closely with the intensive outpatient program to assure adherence to the treatment plan, the status of Mr. Parker's drinking, and coordinate with his cancer providers. After completing intensive outpatient treatment, Mr. Parker initially hoped to "be done" with substance use treatment. The cancer clinic providers encouraged ongoing treatment, and Dr. Freeman used motivational interviewing to enhance readiness to engage in continuing care. As a result, Mr. Parker agreed to engage in continuing care groups every other week with others early in recovery.

After a worsening of his cancer symptoms, Mr. Parker had a return to drinking. Dr. Freeman coordinated with the community substance use treatment program and, in collaboration with Mr. Parker, assisted in helping him receive more intensive continuing care services to provide additional support to his recovery. Mr. Parker initially started with weekly outpatient individual sessions focused on cognitive behavioral skills. After several months of treatment he successfully transitioned back to continuing care groups every other week.

While Dr. Freeman did not serve as Mr. Parker's primary provider, he played a vital role of recognizing decision points where treatment services could be enhanced or decreased to address Mr. Parker's changing needs. Dr. Freeman also played an important role in collaborating with the substance use providers and creating a link between his cancer treatment and the substance use treatment clinic.

10 FUTURE DIRECTION OF PRACTICE

Although it is not an idea we developed—in fact, it is one we have followed—we hope that this book has illustrated the need for clinical health psychologists and other mental health professionals working with medical patients to become more adept at addressing harmful substance use. This chapter focuses on aspects of care delivery that will promote better integration between the psychological and medical care of the medical patient with harmful substance use. We also provide future directions for training in psychology to address this gap in many psychologists' knowledge and skill sets. Finally, we discuss new challenges we foresee on the horizon for providers addressing harmful substance use in medical patients.

ACHIEVING INTEGRATION OF CARE

We believe that integrating care for harmful substance use into medical treatment settings has the potential to dramatically improve prevention, early detection, and intervention for substance use across the spectrum. Although most medical settings will rely on referral to specialty care for

http://dx.doi.org/10.1037/0000160-011
Psychological Treatment of Medical Patients Struggling With Harmful Substance Use, by J. A. Schumacher and D. C. Williams

patients with substance use disorders, an improved referral process, universal screening, and continuing care for patients who complete specialty treatment programs can be achieved in many settings.

Universal Screening

The first and perhaps easiest step toward integrated care is universal screening for all new patients and annual screening for all existing patients. Although there are some telltale signs of harmful substance use, such as repeated requests for early refills on scheduled medications, positive toxicology screening, alcohol on the breath during a visit, track marks from repeated use of intravenous drugs, or signs of intoxication during a visit, in our experience, patients who are engaging in harmful substance use are usually indistinguishable from patients who are not at a typical visit for medical or psychological care. Universal screening increases the chance that harmful substance use will be detected and can be addressed as needed. In most settings, this is best achieved using a process than begins with single-item prescreens for harmful drug and alcohol use embedded with other items completed in the waiting room. Sample prescreening items are included in Chapter 4, Table 4.2. For patients that have been referred for psychological or psychiatric issues, the *DSM–5* Level 1 Cross-Cutting Symptom Measure is a tool available from the American Psychiatric Association (2013b) that enables clinicians to quickly assess signs and symptoms across psychiatric diagnoses, and also includes items to prescreen for harmful alcohol and drug use.

In most settings, the vast majority of patients will screen negative for harmful substance use. In a busy practice setting, negative prescreens may receive no further attention. However, we encourage using this opportunity to affirm low-risk use and encourage patients to continue protecting their health in that way. Positive prescreens are followed by additional questions to help determine problem severity and recommended treatment. Clinicians who are less familiar with substance use disorders may choose to use resources developed by the World Health Organization and the Substance Abuse and Mental Health Services Association to facilitate screening.

USAUDIT: The Alcohol Use Disorders Identification Test, Adapted for Use in the United States: A Guide for Primary Care Practitioners, published by the Substance Abuse and Mental Health Services Administration (Babor et al., 2016), provides in-depth information about screening for harmful alcohol use with the USAUDIT including information about how to determine level of care needed and how to deliver a brief intervention to patients who would benefit from cutting down on their drinking but do not need specialty care. This guide is available online (http://www.ct.gov/dmhas/lib/dmhas/publications/USAUDIT-2017.pdf).

The Alcohol, Smoking and Substance Involvement Screening Test (ASSIST): Manual for Use in Primary Care, published by the World Health Organization (Humeniuk et al., 2010a), provides in-depth information about screening for harmful alcohol, drug, and tobacco use using the ASSIST, including how to determine level of care needed. This guide is available online (http://www.who.int/substance_abuse/activities/assist/en/).

The ASSIST-Linked Brief Intervention for Hazardous and Harmful Substance Use: Manual for Use in Primary Care, published by the World Health Organization (Humeniuk et al., 2010b), can be used with the ASSIST to provide brief intervention for patients who would benefit from making changes in alcohol, tobacco, or drug use but do not need specialty care. This guide is available online (http://www.who.int/substance_abuse/activities/assist/en/).

Screenings for Drug Use in General Medical Settings: A Resource Guide for Providers, produced by the National Institute on Drug Abuse (NIDA), focuses specifically on drug use using a NIDA-modified version of the ASSIST. The intervention follows a 5 A's model: Ask, Advise, Assess, Assist, Arrange. This guide is available online (https://www.drugabuse.gov/sites/default/files/resource_guide.pdf).

For patients who are using drugs or alcohol in ways that place their health at risk but do not yet need specialty care, it is important that all psychologists be prepared to offer brief intervention. Brief intervention is designed to increase awareness and enhance motivation to make changes in substance use. In addition to the information in Chapter 4 of this book, the guides described above are useful tools for clinicians who are uncertain about delivering brief interventions. The Substance Abuse and Mental Health Services Administration also provides numerous resources related to delivery of brief interventions including information on CPT codes for reimbursement (https://www.samhsa.gov/sbirt). Clinicians are also encouraged to get training in motivational interviewing, as this communication style is an important foundation of brief interventions (Miller & Rollnick, 2013).

Treatment Referrals

As outlined in Chapter 4, it is important for clinical health psychologists to become familiar with substance treatment resources in their geographic region, including the intensity (e.g., outpatient, day treatment, residential, detoxification services) and types (e.g., cognitive behavioral, 12 step, contingency management) of treatments offered. This knowledge will help ensure that any referrals patients receive fit their needs and preferences. For patients who will return to your care or continue in your care while they receive specialty substance treatment, it is important to maintain ongoing communication with the substance treatment facility.

Continuing Care

Because substance use disorders are chronic, relapsing conditions (McLellan et al., 2000), any patient who has a history of substance use disorder should receive ongoing monitoring. For some patients this may involve periodically asking about their substance use and affirming them for ongoing low-risk use. For others it may involve planning for how to manage cravings during times that are high risk. When patients do relapse or return to hazardous use, maintaining an ongoing, collaborative relationship is important. Making behavior change is difficult, and sometimes multiple attempts at addressing substance use will be required to help the patient reduce substance risk levels. At these times, negative judgments, using scare tactics, or confrontation can actually push patients away from change and further entrench them in their hazardous use (Miller & Rollnick, 2013). Monitoring our internal reactions to patients and maintaining a stance of respect and worth invites the patient to continue on the path to recovery.

TRAINING THE NEXT GENERATION

It is important for clinical health psychologists involved in training programs to take whatever steps they can to stop the cycle of insufficient knowledge, skills, and confidence in addressing patients with harmful substance use. Our years as faculty in training programs for various types of health-care providers, including psychologists, have made us aware that any implicit or explicit messages trainees receive about substance use disorders not being something most health-care providers can or should address are impactful. In fact, small, off-handed comments during practicum placements can undermine the formal curriculum in profound ways. This is sometimes called the "hidden curriculum" in medical education (Hafferty & Gaufberg, 2017). Thus, at a minimum, all psychologists who interact with trainees should avoid any comments or behaviors that imply things such as the following: substance use disorders are moral failings, providers are too busy to "deal" with those with harmful drug use, or psychologists should not get involved in addressing harmful substance use. Beyond that, psychologists should invite trainees to shadow screening and brief intervention when it is conducted or even encourage trainees to conduct these activities as we do in our training programs. Linkages with outside substance use treatment facilities are another way we have addressed this gap in training. We have formed mutually beneficial relationships between our training programs and multiple community-based substance use treatment programs. Through these linkages, the treatment programs are able to enhance the mental health treatment they can provide and our trainees develop knowledge, skills, and confidence in working with patients with harmful substance use. With the prevalence rates of harmful substance use and the shockingly high rates of co-occurrence of harmful substance use with other psychiatric illnesses, we simply do not have the luxury of not addressing harmful substance use regardless of the treatment setting we work in.

CHALLENGES ON THE HORIZON

The current opioid epidemic should serve as a cautionary tale about the potential dangers of prescribing medications with abuse liability. As we were writing this chapter, we watched a story on the nightly news on the dangers of rising benzodiazepine prescriptions. While the problems our patients face with pain, anxiety, trauma, and more are real and daunting, medications with abuse liability have the potential to create more harm and reduce quality of life by creating addiction-related problems on top of their already complex problems. In addition to cannabis (discussed in Chapter 1), several medications such as these are appearing on the horizon, and we urge caution and restraint. One example is the use of ketamine for depression. While ketamine does have some legitimate medical uses (e.g., anesthesia), ketamine is also a serious drug of abuse (often known as "special K"). There is growing support toward approval of ketamine for the treatment of depression (e.g., Serafini, Howland, Rovedi, Girardi, & Amore, 2014; Xu et al., 2016). While a fast-acting medication to reduce depressive symptomatology would be a major breakthrough in treating mood disorders, we predict that, like opioids, without close regulation of prescribing, there could be major costs associated with its use and a domino effect of secondary problems that will outweigh the benefits. A second is example is 3,4-methylendedioxymethylampheatime (MDMA) as an adjunct to psychotherapy for treatment-refractory PTSD. MDMA, also called "ecstasy" or "molly," is chemically similar to stimulants and hallucinogens and alters mood and perception, and it has been used recreationally by more than 18 million people (National Institute on Drug Abuse, 2017). There is promising evidence that administering MDMA during psychotherapy for PTSD may enhance outcomes for patients who have failed to benefit from prior treatments, and when used as indicated, it is fairly low risk (Sessa, 2011). However, many medications with abuse liability are not prescribed or used as indicated or recommended. Benzodiazepines are typically recommended for durations of no more than a few weeks, but they are often prescribed for months, years, or even decades (Neutel, 2005). It is important for psychologists who are knowledgeable about addictions to help educate prescribers who may be less familiar with the risks of medications with abuse liability about the need for caution. Psychologists and other mental health professionals play a key role in not only addressing hazardous substance use in our patient populations but also in advocating within the scientific and medical communities for treatment options that are most likely to benefit our patients and avoid the negative outcomes of hazardous substance use.

References

Aalto, M., Pekuri, P., & Seppa, K. (2002). Primary health care professionals' activity in intervening in patients' alcohol drinking: A patient perspective. *Drug and Alcohol Dependence, 66*, 39–43. http://dx.doi.org/10.1016/S0376-8716(01)00179-X

Adamson, S. J., Sellman, J. D., & Frampton, C. M. A. (2009). Patient predictors of alcohol treatment outcome: A systematic review. *Journal of Substance Abuse Treatment, 36*, 75–86. http://dx.doi.org/10.1016/j.jsat.2008.05.007

Ahmed, A. T., Karter, A. J., & Liu, J. (2006). Alcohol consumption is inversely associated with adherence to diabetes self-care behaviours. *Diabetic Medicine, 23*, 795–802. http://dx.doi.org/10.1111/j.1464-5491.2006.01878.x

Albert, P. R. (2015). Why is depression more prevalent in women? *Journal of Psychiatry & Neuroscience, 40*, 219–221. http://dx.doi.org/10.1503/jpn.150205

Alcoholics Anonymous. (1952). *Twelve steps and twelve traditions.* Retrieved from https://www.aa.org/pages/en_US/twelve-steps-and-twelve-traditions

Alcoholics Anonymous. (2001). *Big book* (4th ed.). Retrieved from https://www.aa.org/pages/en_US/alcoholics-anonymous

Aldridge, A., Linford, R., & Bray, J. (2017). Substance use outcomes of patients served by a large US implementation of Screening, Brief Intervention and Referral to Treatment (SBIRT). *Addiction, 112*(Suppl. 2), 43–53. http://dx.doi.org/10.1111/add.13651

Alegría, A. A., Hasin, D. S., Nunes, E. V., Liu, S. M., Davies, C., Grant, B. F., & Blanco, C. (2010). Comorbidity of generalized anxiety disorder and substance use disorders: Results from the National Epidemiologic Survey on Alcohol and Related Conditions. *The Journal of Clinical Psychiatry, 71*, 1187–1195. http://dx.doi.org/10.4088/JCP09m05328gry

Allen, J. P., Sillanaukee, P., Strid, N., & Litten, R. Z. (2003). Biomarkers of heavy drinking. In J. P. Allen & V. B. Wilson (Eds.), *Assessing alcohol problems: A guide for clinicians and researchers* (2nd ed., pp. 37–54; NIH Publication No. 03-3745). Bethesda, MD: U.S. Department of Health and Human

Services, Public Health Service, National Institutes of Health, National Institute on Alcohol Abuse and Alcoholism.

American Academy of Family Physicians. (2017). *Summary of recommendations for clinical preventive services* (Order No. 1968). Retrieved from https://www.aafp.org/dam/AAFP/documents/patient_care/clinical_recommendations/cps-recommendations.pdf

American Academy of Sleep Medicine. (2014). *International classification of sleep disorders: Diagnostic and coding manual* (3rd ed.). Darien, IL: Author.

American College of Obstetricians and Gynecologists Committee on Health Care for Underserved Women. (2011). At-risk drinking and alcohol dependence: Obstetric and gynecologic implications (Committee Opinion No. 496). *Obstetrics and Gynecology, 118*, 383–388. http://dx.doi.org/10.1097/AOG.0b013e31822c9906

American Psychiatric Association. (2000). *Diagnostic and statistical manual of mental disorders* (4th ed., text rev.). Washington, DC: Author.

American Psychiatric Association. (2013a). *Diagnostic and statistical manual of mental disorders* (5th ed.). Washington, DC: Author.

American Psychiatric Association. (2013b). DSM–5 *Self-Rated Level 1 Cross-Cutting Symptom Measure, Adult.* Retrieved from https://www.psychiatry.org/psychiatrists/practice/dsm/educational-resources/assessment-measures

American Psychiatric Association, Work Group on Substance Use Disorders. (2006). *Practice guideline for the treatment of patients with substance use disorders.* Retrieved from http://psychiatryonline.org/pb/assets/raw/sitewide/practice_guidelines/guidelines/substanceuse.pdf

Anderson, D. J., McGovern, J. P., & DuPont, R. L. (1999). The origins of the Minnesota Model of addiction treatment—A first person account. *Journal of Addictive Diseases, 18*, 107–114. http://dx.doi.org/10.1300/J069v18n01_10

Anthony, J. C. (2006). The epidemiology of cannabis dependence. In R. A. Roffman & R. S. Stephens (Eds.), *Cannabis dependence: Its nature, consequences and treatment* (pp. 58–105). Cambridge, England: Cambridge University Press. http://dx.doi.org/10.1017/CBO9780511544248.006

Anthony, J. C., Warner, L. A., & Kessler, R. C. (1994). Comparative epidemiology of dependence on tobacco, alcohol, controlled substances and inhalants: Basic findings from the National Comorbidity Survey. *Experimental and Clinical Psychopharmacology, 2*, 244–268. http://dx.doi.org/10.1037/1064-1297.2.3.244

Arnedt, J. T., Conroy, D. A., Armitage, R., & Brower, K. J. (2011). Cognitive-behavioral therapy for insomnia in alcohol dependent patients: A randomized controlled pilot trial. *Behaviour Research and Therapy, 49*, 227–233. http://dx.doi.org/10.1016/j.brat.2011.02.003

Babor, T. F., Del Boca, F., & Bray, J. W. (2017). Screening, brief intervention and referral to treatment: Implications of SAMHSA's SBIRT initiative for substance abuse policy and practice. *Addiction, 112*(Suppl. 2), 110–117. http://dx.doi.org/10.1111/add.13675

Babor, T. F., Higgins-Biddle, J. C., Dauser, D., Burleson, J. A., Zarkin, G. A., & Bray, J. (2006, November–December). Brief interventions for at-risk drinking: Patient outcomes and cost-effectiveness in managed care organizations. *Alcohol and Alcoholism, 41,* 624–631. http://dx.doi.org/10.1093/alcalc/agl078

Babor, T. F., Higgins-Biddle, J. C., & Saunders, J. B. (2016). *USAUDIT: The Alcohol Use Disorders Identification Test, Adapted for Use in the United States: A guide for primary care practitioners.* Rockville, MD: Substance Abuse and Mental Health Services Administration. Retrieved from http://www.ct.gov/dmhas/lib/dmhas/publications/USAUDIT-2017.pdf

Babson, K. A., Boden, M. T., Harris, A. H., Stickle, T. R., & Bonn-Miller, M. O. (2013). Poor sleep quality as a risk factor for lapse following a cannabis quit attempt. *Journal of Substance Abuse Treatment, 44,* 438–443. http://dx.doi.org/10.1016/j.jsat.2012.08.224

Baker, A. L., Kavanagh, D. J., Kay-Lambkin, F. J., Hunt, S. A., Lewin, T. J., Carr, V. J., & McElduff, P. (2014). Randomized controlled trial of MICBT for co-existing alcohol misuse and depression: Outcomes to 36-months. *Journal of Substance Abuse Treatment, 46,* 281–290. http://dx.doi.org/10.1016/j.jsat.2013.10.001

Baker, A. L., Thornton, L. K., Hiles, S., Hides, L., & Lubman, D. I. (2012). Psychological interventions for alcohol misuse among people with co-occurring depression or anxiety disorders: A systematic review. *Journal of Affective Disorders, 139,* 217–229. http://dx.doi.org/10.1016/j.jad.2011.08.004

Banks, S., & Dinges, D. F. (2007). Behavioral and physiological consequences of sleep restriction. *Journal of Clinical Sleep Medicine, 3,* 519–528.

Barbosa, C., Cowell, A., Bray, J., & Aldridge, A. (2015). The cost-effectiveness of alcohol screening, brief intervention, and referral to treatment (SBIRT) in emergency and outpatient medical settings. *Journal of Substance Abuse Treatment, 53,* 1–8. http://dx.doi.org/10.1016/j.jsat.2015.01.003

Barclay, J. S., Owens, J. E., & Blackhall, L. J. (2014). Screening for substance abuse risk in cancer patients using the Opioid Risk Tool and urine drug screen. *Supportive Care in Cancer, 22,* 1883–1888. http://dx.doi.org/10.1007/s00520-014-2167-6

Bastien, C. H., Vallières, A., & Morin, C. M. (2001). Validation of the Insomnia Severity Index as an outcome measure for insomnia research. *Sleep Medicine, 2,* 297–307. http://dx.doi.org/10.1016/S1389-9457(00)00065-4

Beattie, M. C., & Longabaugh, R. (1999). General and alcohol-specific social support following treatment. *Addictive Behaviors, 24,* 593–606. http://dx.doi.org/10.1016/S0306-4603(98)00120-8

Beck, A. K., Forbes, E., Baker, A. L., Kelly, P. J., Deane, F. P., Shakeshaft, A., . . . Kelly, J. F. (2017). Systematic review of SMART Recovery: Outcomes, process variables, and implications for research. *Psychology of Addictive Behaviors, 31,* 1–20. http://dx.doi.org/10.1037/adb0000237

Beck, A. T., Steer, R. A., & Brown, G. K. (1996). *BDI–II: Beck Depression Inventory: Manual* (2nd ed.). San Antonio, TX: Psychological Corporation.

Bedard-Gilligan, M., Kaysen, D., Desai, S., & Lee, C. M. (2011). Alcohol-involved assault: Associations with posttrauma alcohol use, consequences, and expectancies. *Addictive Behaviors, 36,* 1076–1082. http://dx.doi.org/10.1016/j.addbeh.2011.07.001

Bien, T. H., Miller, W. R., & Tonigan, J. S. (1993). Brief interventions for alcohol problems: A review. *Addiction, 88,* 315–336. http://dx.doi.org/10.1111/j.1360-0443.1993.tb00820.x

Black, D. W., & Andreasen, N. C. (2014). *Introductory textbook of psychiatry* (6th ed.). Arlington, VA: American Psychiatric Publishing.

Blanco, C., Alegría, A. A., Liu, S. M., Secades-Villa, R., Sugaya, L., Davies, C., & Nunes, E. V. (2012). Differences among major depressive disorder with and without co-occurring substance use disorders and substance-induced depressive disorder: Results from the National Epidemiologic Survey on Alcohol and Related Conditions. *The Journal of Clinical Psychiatry, 73,* 865–873. http://dx.doi.org/10.4088/JCP.10m06673

Blevins, C. A., Weathers, F. W., Davis, M. T., Witte, T. K., & Domino, J. L. (2015). The Posttraumatic Stress Disorder Checklist for *DSM-5* (PCL-5): Development and initial psychometric evaluation. *Journal of Traumatic Stress, 28,* 489–498. http://dx.doi.org/10.1002/jts.22059

Blodgett, J. C., Maisel, N. C., Fuh, I. L., Wilbourne, P. L., & Finney, J. W. (2014). How effective is continuing care for substance use disorders? A meta-analytic review. *Journal of Substance Abuse Treatment, 46,* 87–97. http://dx.doi.org/10.1016/j.jsat.2013.08.022

Bolton, J. M., Robinson, J., & Sareen, J. (2009). Self-medication of mood disorders with alcohol and drugs in the National Epidemiologic Survey on Alcohol and Related Conditions. *Journal of Affective Disorders, 115,* 367–375. http://dx.doi.org/10.1016/j.jad.2008.10.003

Breslow, R. A., Dong, C., & White, A. (2015). Prevalence of alcohol-interactive prescription medication use among current drinkers: United States, 1999 to 2010. *Alcoholism: Clinical and Experimental Research, 39,* 371–379. http://dx.doi.org/10.1111/acer.12633

Brower, K. J. (2015). Assessment and treatment of insomnia in adult patients with alcohol use disorders. *Alcohol, 49,* 417–427. http://dx.doi.org/10.1016/j.alcohol.2014.12.003

Brower, K. J., Aldrich, M. S., Robinson, E. A. R., Zucker, R. A., & Greden, J. F. (2001). Insomnia, self-medication, and relapse to alcoholism. *The American Journal of Psychiatry, 158,* 399–404. http://dx.doi.org/10.1176/appi.ajp.158.3.399

Brown, R. L., Dimond, A. R., Hulisz, D., Saunders, L. A., & Bobula, J. A. (2007). Pharmacoepidemiology of potential alcohol-prescription drug interactions among primary care patients with alcohol-use disorders. *Journal of the*

American Pharmacists Association, 47, 135–139. http://dx.doi.org/10.1331/ XWH7-R0X8-1817-8N2L

Brown, R. L., Leonard, T., Saunders, L. A., & Papasouliotis, O. (2001). A two-item conjoint screen for alcohol and other drug problems. *The Journal of the American Board of Family Practice, 14*(2), 95–106.

Brown, S. A., Irwin, M., & Schuckit, M. A. (1991). Changes in anxiety among abstinent male alcoholics. *Journal of Studies on Alcohol, 52*, 55–61. http://dx.doi.org/10.15288/jsa.1991.52.55

Brown, S. A., & Schuckit, M. A. (1988). Changes in depression among abstinent alcoholics. *Journal of Studies on Alcohol, 49*, 412–417. http://dx.doi.org/10.15288/jsa.1988.49.412

Buckner, J. D., Bonn-Miller, M. O., Zvolensky, M. J., & Schmidt, N. B. (2007). Marijuana use motives and social anxiety among marijuana-using young adults. *Addictive Behaviors, 32*, 2238–2252. http://dx.doi.org/10.1016/j.addbeh.2007.04.004

Buckner, J. D., Schmidt, N. B., Lang, A. R., Small, J. W., Schlauch, R. C., & Lewinsohn, P. M. (2008). Specificity of social anxiety disorder as a risk factor for alcohol and cannabis dependence. *Journal of Psychiatric Research, 42*, 230–239. http://dx.doi.org/10.1016/j.jpsychires.2007.01.002

Bush, K., Kivlahan, D. R., McDonell, M. B., Fihn, S. D., & Bradley, K. A. (1998). The AUDIT alcohol consumption questions (AUDIT-C): An effective brief screening test for problem drinking. *Archives of Internal Medicine, 158*, 1789–1795. http://dx.doi.org/10.1001/archinte.158.16.1789

Buysse, D. J., Reynolds, C. F., III, Monk, T. H., Berman, S. R., & Kupfer, D. J. (1989). The Pittsburgh Sleep Quality Index (PSQI): A new instrument for psychiatric research and practice. *Psychiatry Research, 28*, 193–213. http://dx.doi.org/10.1016/0165-1781(89)90047-4

Canfield, M. C., Keller, C. E., Frydrych, L. M., Ashrafioun, L., Purdy, C. H., & Blondell, R. D. (2010). Prescription opioid use among patients seeking treatment for opioid dependence. *Journal of Addiction Medicine, 4*, 108–113. http://dx.doi.org/10.1097/ADM.0b013e3181b5a713

Capaldi, D. M., Knoble, N. B., Shortt, J. W., & Kim, H. K. (2012). A systematic review of risk factors for intimate partner violence. *Partner Abuse, 3*, 231–280. http://dx.doi.org/10.1891/1946-6560.3.2.231

Center for Behavioral Health Statistics and Quality. (2016). *2015 National Survey on Drug Use and Health: Detailed table.* Rockville, MD: Substance Abuse and Mental Health Services Association. Retrieved from https://www.samhsa.gov/data/sites/default/files/NSDUH-DetTabs-2015/NSDUH-DetTabs-2015/NSDUH-DetTabs-2015.pdf

Chan, Y.-F., Huang, H., Bradley, K., & Unützer, J. (2014). Referral for substance abuse treatment and depression improvement among patients with co-occurring disorders seeking behavioral health services in primary care.

Journal of Substance Abuse Treatment, 46, 106–112. http://dx.doi.org/10.1016/j.jsat.2013.08.016

Chi, F. W., Weisner, C. M., Mertens, J. R., Ross, T. B., & Sterling, S. A. (2017). Alcohol brief intervention in primary care: Blood pressure outcomes in hypertensive patients. *Journal of Substance Abuse Treatment, 77*, 45–51. http://dx.doi.org/10.1016/j.jsat.2017.03.009

Cicero, T. J., & Ellis, M. S. (2017). Understanding the demand side of the prescription opioid epidemic: Does the initial source of opioids matter? *Drug and Alcohol Dependence, 173*(Suppl. 1), S4–S10. http://dx.doi.org/10.1016/j.drugalcdep.2016.03.014

Cicero, T. J., Ellis, M. S., Surratt, H. L., & Kurtz, S. P. (2014). The changing face of heroin use in the United States: A retrospective analysis of the past 50 years. *JAMA: Psychiatry, 71*, 821–826. http://dx.doi.org/10.1001/jamapsychiatry.2014.366

Coffey, S. F., Schumacher, J. A., Brady, K. T., & Cotton, B. D. (2007). Changes in PTSD symptomatology during acute and protracted alcohol and cocaine abstinence. *Drug and Alcohol Dependence, 87*, 241–248. http://dx.doi.org/10.1016/j.drugalcdep.2006.08.025

Coffey, S. F., Schumacher, J. A., Nosen, E., Littlefield, A. K., Henslee, A. M., Lappen, A., & Stasiewicz, P. R. (2016). Trauma-focused exposure therapy for chronic posttraumatic stress disorder in alcohol and drug dependent patients: A randomized controlled trial. *Psychology of Addictive Behaviors, 30*(7), 778–790. http://dx.doi.org/10.1037/adb0000201

Conca, A. J., & Worthen, D. R. (2012). Nonprescription drug abuse. *Journal of Pharmacy Practice, 25*, 13–21. http://dx.doi.org/10.1177/0897190011431148

Conner, K. R., Pinquart, M., & Gamble, S. A. (2009). Meta-analysis of depression and substance use among individuals with alcohol use disorders. *Journal of Substance Abuse Treatment, 37*, 127–137. http://dx.doi.org/10.1016/j.jsat.2008.11.007

Copello, A. G., Velleman, R. D. B., & Templeton, L. J. (2005). Family interventions in the treatment of alcohol and drug problems. *Drug and Alcohol Review, 24*, 369–385. http://dx.doi.org/10.1080/09595230500302356

Costanzo, S., Di Castelnuovo, A., Donati, M. B., Iacoviello, L., & de Gaetano, G. (2010). Alcohol consumption and mortality in patients with cardiovascular disease: A meta-analysis. *Journal of the American College of Cardiology, 55*, 1339–1347. http://dx.doi.org/10.1016/j.jacc.2010.01.006

Crews, F., He, J., & Hodge, C. (2007). Adolescent cortical development: A critical period of vulnerability for addiction. *Pharmacology, Biochemistry and Behavior, 86*, 189–199. http://dx.doi.org/10.1016/j.pbb.2006.12.001

Currie, S. R., Clark, S., Hodgins, D. C., & El-Guebaly, N. (2004). Randomized controlled trial of brief cognitive–behavioural interventions for insomnia in recovering alcoholics. *Addiction, 99*, 1121–1132. http://dx.doi.org/10.1111/j.1360-0443.2004.00835.x

Currie, S. R., Clark, S., Rimac, S., & Malhotra, S. (2003). Comprehensive assessment of insomnia in recovering alcoholics using daily sleep diaries and ambulatory monitoring. *Alcoholism: Clinical and Experimental Research, 27,* 1262–1269. http://dx.doi.org/10.1097/01.ALC.0000081622.03973.57

D'Amico, E. J., Paddock, S. M., Burnam, A., & Kung, F. Y. (2005). Identification of and guidance for problem drinking by general medical providers: Results from a national survey. *Medical Care, 43,* 229–236. http://www.jstor.org/stable/3768221. http://dx.doi.org/10.1097/00005650-200503000-00005

Davis, L. L., Frazier, E., Husain, M. M., Warden, D., Trivedi, M., Fava, M., . . . Rush, A. J. (2006). Substance use disorder comorbidity in major depressive disorder: A confirmatory analysis of the STAR*D cohort. *The American Journal on Addictions, 15,* 278–285. http://dx.doi.org/10.1080/10550490600754317

Dev, R., Parsons, H. A., Palla, S., Palmer, J. L., Del Fabbro, E., & Bruera, E. (2011). Undocumented alcoholism and its correlation with tobacco and illegal drug use in advanced cancer patients. *Cancer, 117,* 4551–4556. http://dx.doi.org/10.1002/cncr.26082

Dimidjian, S., Barrera, M., Jr., Martell, C., Muñoz, R. F., & Lewinsohn, P. M. (2011). The origins and current status of behavioral activation treatments for depression. *Annual Review of Clinical Psychology, 7,* 1–38. http://dx.doi.org/10.1146/annurev-clinpsy-032210-104535

Dimoff, J. D., Sayette, M. A., & Norcross, J. C. (2017). Addiction training in clinical psychology: Are we keeping up with the rising epidemic? *American Psychologist, 72,* 689–695. http://dx.doi.org/10.1037/amp0000140

Donoghue, K., Elzerbi, C., Saunders, R., Whittington, C., Pilling, S., & Drummond, C. (2015). The efficacy of acamprosate and naltrexone in the treatment of alcohol dependence, Europe versus the rest of the world: A meta-analysis. *Addiction, 110,* 920–930. http://dx.doi.org/10.1111/add.12875

Dowell, D., Haegerich, T. M., & Chou, R. (2016). CDC guideline for prescribing opioids for chronic pain—United States, 2016. *Morbidity and Mortality Weekly Report, 65*(No. RR-1). Advance online publication. Retrieved from https://www.cdc.gov/mmwr/volumes/65/rr/rr6501e1.htm

Drug Enforcement Agency. (2017). *Drugs of abuse: A DEA resource guide.* Retrieved from https://www.dea.gov/pr/multimedia-library/publications/drug_of_abuse.pdf

Dworkin, E. R., Zambrano-Vazquez, L., Cunningham, S. R., Pittenger, S. L., Schumacher, J. A., Stasiewicz, P. R., & Coffey, S. F. (2017). Treating PTSD in pregnant and postpartum rural women with substance use disorders. *Journal of Rural Mental Health, 41,* 136–151. http://dx.doi.org/10.1037/rmh0000057

Edinger, J. D., & Carney, C. E. (2008). *Overcoming insomnia: A cognitive-behavioral therapy approach* [Workbook]. New York, NY: Oxford University Press.

Ewing, J. A. (1984). Detecting alcoholism. The CAGE questionnaire. *JAMA, 252*, 1905–1907. http://dx.doi.org/10.1001/jama.1984.03350140051025

Fairholme, C. P., Nosen, E. L., Nillni, Y. I., Schumacher, J. A., Tull, M. T., & Coffey, S. F. (2013). Sleep disturbance and emotion dysregulation as trans-diagnostic processes in a comorbid sample. *Behaviour Research and Therapy, 51*, 540–546. http://dx.doi.org/10.1016/j.brat.2013.05.014

Falk, D. E., Yi, H.-Y., & Hilton, M. E. (2008). Age of onset and temporal sequencing of lifetime *DSM–IV* alcohol use disorders relative to comorbid mood and anxiety disorders. *Drug and Alcohol Dependence, 94*, 234–245. http://dx.doi.org/10.1016/j.drugalcdep.2007.11.022

Fishman, M. J., Shulman, G. D., Mee-Lee, D., Kolodner, G., & Wilford, B. B. (2010). *ASAM patient placement criteria: Supplement on pharmacotherapies for alcohol use disorders*. Philadelphia, PA: Lippincott Williams & Wilkins.

Fletcher, A. M. (2013). *Inside rehab: The surprising truth about addiction treatment—And how to get help that works*. New York, NY: Penguin Group.

Friedrich, M. J. (2017). Depression is the leading cause of disability around the world. *Journal of the American Medical Association, 317*, 1517. http://dx.doi.org/10.1001/jama.2017.3826

Foa, E. B., Yusko, D. A., McLean, C. P., Suvak, M. K., Bux, D. A., Jr., Oslin, D., . . . Volpicelli, J. (2013). Concurrent naltrexone and prolonged exposure therapy for patients with comorbid alcohol dependence and PTSD: A randomized clinical trial. *JAMA, 310*, 488–495. http://dx.doi.org/10.1001/jama.2013.8268

Ghuran, A., & Nolan, J. (2000). The cardiac complications of recreational drug use. *The Western Journal of Medicine, 173*, 412–415. http://dx.doi.org/10.1136/ewjm.173.6.412

Glass, J. E., Hamilton, A. M., Powell, B. J., Perron, B. E., Brown, R. T., & Ilgen, M. A. (2015). Specialty substance use disorder services following brief alcohol intervention: A meta-analysis of randomized controlled trials. *Addiction, 110*, 1404–1415. http://dx.doi.org/10.1111/add.12950

Grant, B. F., Chou, S. P., Saha, T. D., Pickering, R. P., Kerridge, B. T., Ruan, W. J., . . . Hasin, D. S. (2017). Prevalence of 12-month alcohol use, high-risk drinking, and *DSM–IV* alcohol use disorder in the United States, 2001–2002 to 2012–2013: Results from the National Epidemiologic Survey on Alcohol and Related Conditions. *JAMA Psychiatry, 74*, 911–923. http://dx.doi.org/10.1001/jamapsychiatry.2017.2161

Grant, B. F., Goldstein, R. B., Saha, T. D., Chou, S. P., Jung, J., Zhang, H., . . . Hasin, D. S. (2015). Epidemiology of *DSM–5* alcohol use disorder: Results from the National Epidemiologic Survey on Alcohol and Related Conditions III. *JAMA Psychiatry, 72*, 757–766. http://dx.doi.org/10.1001/jamapsychiatry.2015.0584

Grant, B. F., Saha, T. D., Ruan, W. J., Goldstein, R. B., Chou, S. P., Jung, J., . . . Hasin, D. S. (2016). Epidemiology of *DSM–5* Drug Use Disorder: Results from the National Epidemiologic Survey on Alcohol and Related Conditions-III. *JAMA Psychiatry, 73*, 39–47. http://dx.doi.org/10.1001/jamapsychiatry.2015.2132

Grant, B. F., Stinson, F. S., Dawson, D. A., Chou, S. P., Dufour, M. C., Compton, W., . . . Kaplan, K. (2004). Prevalence and co-occurrence of substance use disorders and mood and anxiety disorders. *Archives of General Psychiatry, 61*, 807–817. http://dx.doi.org/10.1001/archpsyc.61.8.807

Greenfield, S. F., Back, S. E., Lawson, K., & Brady, K. T. (2010). Substance abuse in women. *Psychiatric Clinics of North America, 33*, 339–355. http://dx.doi.org/10.1016/j.psc.2010.01.004

Greenfield, S. F., Brooks, A. J., Gordon, S. M., Green, C. A., Kropp, F., McHugh, R. K., . . . Miele, G. M. (2007). Substance abuse treatment entry, retention, and outcome in women: A review of the literature. *Drug and Alcohol Dependence, 86*, 1–21. http://dx.doi.org/10.1016/j.drugalcdep.2006.05.012

Grunbaum, J. A., Kann, L., Kinchen, S., Ross, J., Hawkins, J., Lowry, R., . . . Collins, J. (2004). Youth risk behavior surveillance United States, 2003. *Morbidity and Mortality Weekly Report Surveillance Summaries*. Atlanta, GA: Centers for Disease Control and Prevention. Retrieved from http://www.cdc.gov/mmwr/preview/mmwrhtml/ss5302a1.htm

Guydish, J., Werdegar, D., Sorensen, J. L., Clark, W., & Acampora, A. (1998). Drug abuse day treatment: A randomized clinical trial comparing day and residential treatment programs. *Journal of Consulting and Clinical Psychology, 66*, 280–289. http://dx.doi.org/10.1037/0022-006X.66.2.280

Hafferty, F. W., & Gaufberg, E. H. (2017). The hidden curriculum. In J. Dent, R. M. Harden, & D. Hunt (Eds.), *A practical guide for medical teachers* (5th ed., pp. 35–41). New York, NY: Elsevier Health.

Hall, W., & Degenhardt, L. (2009). Adverse health effects of non-medical cannabis use. *The Lancet, 374*, 1383–1391. http://dx.doi.org/10.1016/S0140-6736(09)61037-0

Hargraves, D., White, C., Frederick, R., Cinibulk, M., Peters, M., Young, A., & Elder, N. (2017). Implementing SBIRT (Screening, Brief Intervention and Referral to Treatment) in primary care: Lessons learned from a multi-practice evaluation portfolio. *Public Health Reviews, 38*, 31. http://dx.doi.org/10.1186/s40985-017-0077-0

Harvey, A. G., Murray, G., Chandler, R. A., & Soehner, A. (2011). Sleep disturbance as transdiagnostic: Consideration of neurobiological mechanisms. *Clinical Psychology Review, 31*, 225–235. http://dx.doi.org/10.1016/j.cpr.2010.04.003

Hasin, D. S., & Grant, B. F. (2015). The National Epidemiologic Survey on Alcohol and Related Conditions (NESARC) Waves 1 and 2: Review and summary of findings. *Social Psychiatry and Psychiatric Epidemiology, 50*, 1609–1640. http://dx.doi.org/10.1007/s00127-015-1088-0

Hasin, D. S., O'Brien, C. P., Auriacombe, M., Borges, G., Bucholz, K., Budney, A., . . . Grant, B. F. (2013). *DSM–5* criteria for substance use disorders: Recommendations and rationale. *The American Journal of Psychiatry, 170*, 834–851. http://dx.doi.org/10.1176/appi.ajp.2013.12060782

Hasin, D. S., Saha, T. D., Kerridge, B. T., Goldstein, R. B., Chou, S. P., Zhang, H., . . . Grant, B. F. (2015). Prevalence of marijuana use disorders in the United States between 2001–2002 and 2012–2013. *JAMA Psychiatry*, *72*, 1235–1242. http://dx.doi.org/10.1001/jamapsychiatry.2015.1858

Hasin, D. S., Stinson, F. S., Ogburn, E., & Grant, B. F. (2007). Prevalence, correlates, disability, and comorbidity of *DSM–IV* alcohol abuse and dependence in the United States: Results from the National Epidemiologic Survey on Alcohol and Related Conditions. *Archives of General Psychiatry*, *64*, 830–842. http://dx.doi.org/10.1001/archpsyc.64.7.830

Hasin, D. S., Trautman, K. D., Miele, G. M., Samet, S., Smith, M., & Endicott, J. (1996). Psychiatric Research Interview for Substance and Mental Disorders (PRISM): Reliability for substance abusers. *The American Journal of Psychiatry*, *153*, 1195–1201. http://dx.doi.org/10.1176/ajp.153.9.1195

Hedegaard, H., Warner, M., & Miniño, A. M. (2017). *Drug overdose deaths in the United States, 1999–2016* (NCHS Data Brief No. 294). Hyattsville, MD: National Center for Health Statistics. Retrieved from https://www.cdc.gov/nchs/data/databriefs/db294.pdf

Heinz, A. J., de Wit, H., Lilje, T. C., & Kassel, J. D. (2013). The combined effects of alcohol, caffeine, and expectancies on subjective experience, impulsivity, and risk-taking. *Experimental and Clinical Psychopharmacology*, *21*, 222–234. http://dx.doi.org/10.1037/a0032337

Helander, A., Böttcher, M., Fehr, C., Dahmen, N., & Beck, O. (2009). Detection times for urinary ethyl glucuronide and ethyl sulfate in heavy drinkers during alcohol detoxification. *Alcohol and Alcoholism*, *44*(1), 55–61. http://dx.doi.org/10.1093/alcalc/agn084

Henninger, A., & Sung, H.-E. (2013). History of substance abuse treatment. In G. Bruinsma & D. Weisburd (Eds.), *Encyclopedia of criminology and criminal justice* (pp. 2257–2269). New York, NY: Springer.

Hingson, R., & White, A. (2014). New research findings since the 2007 Surgeon General's call to action to prevent and reduce underage drinking: A review. *Journal of Studies on Alcohol and Drugs*, *75*, 158–169. http://dx.doi.org/10.15288/jsad.2014.75.158

Hofmann, S. G., Sawyer, A. T., Witt, A. A., & Oh, D. (2010). The effect of mindfulness-based therapy on anxiety and depression: A meta-analytic review. *Journal of Consulting and Clinical Psychology*, *78*, 169–183. http://dx.doi.org/10.1037/a0018555

Hruska, B., & Delahanty, D. L. (2012). Application of the stressor vulnerability model to understanding posttraumatic stress disorder (PTSD) and alcohol-related problems in an undergraduate population. *Psychology of Addictive Behaviors*, *26*, 734–746. http://dx.doi.org/10.1037/a0027584

Hughes, T. L., & Eliason, M. (2002). Substance use and abuse in lesbian, gay, bisexual, and transgender populations. *The Journal of Primary Prevention*, *22*, 263–298. http://dx.doi.org/10.1023/A:1013669705086

Humeniuk, R. E., Henry-Edwards, S., Ali, R. L., Poznyak, V., & Monteiro, M. (2010a). *The Alcohol, Smoking and Substance Involvement Screening Test (ASSIST): Manual for use in primary care.* Geneva, Switzerland: World Health Organization.

Humeniuk, R. E., Henry-Edwards, S., Ali, R. L., Poznyak, V., & Monteiro, M. (2010b). *The ASSIST-linked brief intervention for hazardous and harmful substance use: Manual for use in primary care.* Geneva, Switzerland: World Health Organization.

Humphreys, K. (2004). *Circles of recovery: Self-help organizations for addictions.* Cambridge, England: Cambridge University Press.

Institute of Medicine. (2006). *Sleep disorders and sleep deprivation: An unmet public health problem.* Washington, DC: National Academies Press. Retrieved from https://www.nap.edu/catalog/11617/sleep-disorders-and-sleep-deprivation-an-unmet-public-health-problem

Kadden, R., Carroll, K., Donovan, D., Conney, N., Monti, P., Abrams, D., . . . Hester, R. (2003). Cognitive-behavioral coping skills therapy manual: A clinical research guide for therapists treating individuals with alcohol abuse and dependence. In M. E. Mattson (Series Ed.), *Project MATCH Monograph Series* (Vol. 3, NIH Publication No. 94-3724). Rockville, MD: National Institute on Alcohol Abuse and Alcoholism. Retrieved from https://pubs.niaaa.nih.gov/publications/ProjectMatch/match03.pdf

Kay-Lambkin, F., Baker, A., Hunt, S., Kavanagh, D., & Bucci, S. (2005). *Depression and Alcohol Integrated and Single focused Interventions (DAISI): A treatment manual.* Callaghan, NSW, Australia: The University of Newcastle.

Kaysen, D., Dillworth, T. M., Simpson, T., Waldrop, A., Larimer, M. E., & Resick, P. A. (2007). Domestic violence and alcohol use: Trauma-related symptoms and motives for drinking. *Addictive Behaviors, 32,* 1272–1283. http://dx.doi.org/10.1016/j.addbeh.2006.09.007

Kaysen, D., Schumm, J., Pedersen, E. R., Seim, R. W., Bedard-Gilligan, M., & Chard, K. (2014). Cognitive processing therapy for veterans with comorbid PTSD and alcohol use disorders. *Addictive Behaviors, 39,* 420–427. http://dx.doi.org/10.1016/j.addbeh.2013.08.016

Khazaal, Y., Chatton, A., Monney, G., Nallet, A., Khan, R., Zullino, D., & Etter, J.-F. (2015). Internal consistency and measurement equivalence of the cannabis screening questions on the paper-and-pencil face-to-face ASSIST versus the online instrument. *Substance Abuse Treatment, Prevention, and Policy, 10,* 8. http://dx.doi.org/10.1186/s13011-015-0002-9

Khoury, B., Lecomte, T., Fortin, G., Masse, M., Therien, P., Bouchard, V., . . . Hofmann, S. G. (2013). Mindfulness-based therapy: A comprehensive meta-analysis. *Clinical Psychology Review, 33,* 763–771. http://dx.doi.org/10.1016/j.cpr.2013.05.005

King, A. P., Erickson, T. M., Giardino, N. D., Favorite, T., Rauch, S. A., Robinson, E., . . . Liberzon, I. (2013). A pilot study of group mindfulness-based cognitive therapy (MBCT) for combat veterans with posttraumatic stress disorder (PTSD). *Depression and Anxiety, 30,* 638–645. http://dx.doi.org/10.1002/da.22104

Kissin, W., McLeod, C., & McKay, J. (2003). The longitudinal relationship between self-help group attendance and course of recovery. *Evaluation and Program Planning, 26,* 311–323. http://dx.doi.org/10.1016/S0149-7189(03)00035-1

Kranzler, H. R., & Soyka, M. (2018). Diagnosis and pharmacotherapy of alcohol use disorder: A review. *JAMA, 320,* 815–824. http://dx.doi.org/10.1001/jama.2018.11406

Kroenke, K., Spitzer, R. L., & Williams, J. B. (2001). The PHQ–9: Validity of a brief depression severity measure. *Journal of General Internal Medicine, 16,* 606–613. http://dx.doi.org/10.1046/j.1525-1497.2001.016009606.x

Lash, S. J., Burden, J. L., Parker, J. D., Stephens, R. S., Budney, A. J., Horner, R. D., . . . Grambow, S. C. (2013). Contracting, prompting and reinforcing substance use disorder continuing care. *Journal of Substance Abuse Treatment, 44,* 449–456. http://dx.doi.org/10.1016/j.jsat.2012.09.008

Lash, S. J., Stephens, R. S., Burden, J. L., Grambow, S. C., DeMarce, J. M., Jones, M. E., . . . Horner, R. D. (2007). Contracting, prompting, and reinforcing substance use disorder continuing care: A randomized clinical trial. *Psychology of Addictive Behaviors, 21,* 387–397. http://dx.doi.org/10.1037/0893-164X.21.3.387

Lazareck, S., Robinson, J. A., Crum, R. M., Mojtabai, R., Sareen, J., & Bolton, J. M. (2012). A longitudinal investigation of the role of self-medication in the development of comorbid mood and drug use disorders: Findings from the National Epidemiologic Survey on Alcohol and Related Conditions (NESARC). *The Journal of Clinical Psychiatry, 73,* e588–e593. http://dx.doi.org/10.4088/JCP.11m07345

Lee, J. S., Hu, H. M., Edelman, A. L., Brummett, C. M., Englesbe, M. J., Waljee, J. F., . . . Dossett, L. A. (2017). New persistent opioid use among patients with cancer after curative-intent surgery. *Journal of Clinical Oncology, 35,* 4042–4049. http://dx.doi.org/10.1200/JCO.2017.74.1363

Levy, S., Williams, J. F., & American Academy of Pediatrics Committee on Substance Use and Prevention. (2016). Substance use screening, brief intervention, and referral to treatment. *Pediatrics, 138.* Retrieved from http://pediatrics.aappublications.org/content/138/1/e20161211

Li, M. D., & Burmeister, M. (2009). New insights into the genetics of addiction. *Nature Reviews: Genetics, 10,* 225–231. http://dx.doi.org/10.1038/nrg2536

Lichstein, K. L., Durrence, H. H., Taylor, D. J., Bush, A. J., & Riedel, B. W. (2003). Quantitative criteria for insomnia. *Behaviour Research and Therapy, 41,* 427–445. http://dx.doi.org/10.1016/S0005-7967(02)00023-2

Lichstein, K. L., Nau, S. D., Wilson, N. M., Aguillard, R. N., Lester, K. W., Bush, A. J., & McCrae, C. S. (2013). Psychological treatment of hypnotic-dependent insomnia in a primarily older adult sample. *Behaviour Research and Therapy, 51,* 787–796. http://dx.doi.org/10.1016/j.brat.2013.09.006

Lipari, R. N., Ahrnsbrak, R. D., Pemberton, M. R., & Porter, J. D. (2017). Risk and protective factors and estimates of substance use initiation: Results from the 2016 National Survey on Drug Use and Health. *NSDUH Data Review.* Retrieved from https://www.samhsa.gov/data/sites/default/files/NSDUH-DR-FFR3-2016/NSDUH-DR-FFR3-2016.htm

Litt, M. D., Kadden, R. M., Kabela-Cormier, E., & Petry, N. M. (2009). Changing network support for drinking: Network support project 2-year follow-up. *Journal of Consulting and Clinical Psychology, 77,* 229–242. http://dx.doi.org/10.1037/a0015252

Madras, B. K., Compton, W. M., Avula, D., Stegbauer, T., Stein, J. B., & Clark, H. W. (2009). Screening, brief interventions, referral to treatment (SBIRT) for illicit drug and alcohol use at multiple healthcare sites: Comparison at intake and 6 months later. *Drug and Alcohol Dependence, 99,* 280–295. http://dx.doi.org/10.1016/j.drugalcdep.2008.08.003

Madson, M. B., Bethea, A. R., Daniel, S., & Necaise, H. (2008). The state of substance abuse treatment training in counseling and counseling psychology programs: What is and is not happening. *Journal of Teaching in the Addictions, 7,* 164–178. http://dx.doi.org/10.1080/15332700802269177

Mahfoud, Y., Talih, F., Streem, D., & Budur, K. (2009). Sleep disorders in substance abusers: How common are they? *Psychiatry, 6,* 38–42.

Manzoni, G. M., Pagnini, F., Castelnuovo, G., & Molinari, E. (2008). Relaxation training for anxiety: A ten-years systematic review with meta-analysis. *BMC Psychiatry, 8,* 41. http://dx.doi.org/10.1186/1471-244X-8-41

Marcenko, M. O., Kemp, S. P., & Larson, N. C. (2000). Childhood experiences of abuse, later substance use, and parenting outcomes among low-income mothers. *American Journal of Orthopsychiatry, 70,* 316–326. http://dx.doi.org/10.1037/h0087853

Marsh, J. C., Cao, D., Guerrero, E., & Shin, H.-C. (2009). Need-service matching in substance abuse treatment: Racial/ethnic differences. *Evaluation and Program Planning, 32,* 43–51. http://dx.doi.org/10.1016/j.evalprogplan.2008.09.003

Marshall, J. (2008). Medical management of co-morbid anxiety and substance use disorder. In S. H. Stewart & P. J. Conrod (Eds.), *Anxiety and substance use disorders: The vicious cycle of comorbidity* (pp. 221–236). New York, NY: Springer. http://dx.doi.org/10.1007/978-0-387-74290-8_12

Martin, J. L., Burrow-Sánchez, J. J., Iwamoto, D. K., Glidden-Tracey, C. E., & Vaughan, E. L. (2016). Counseling psychology and substance use: Implications for training, practice, and research. *The Counseling Psychologist, 44,* 1106–1126. http://dx.doi.org/10.1177/0011000016667536

Martin, S. L., Beaumont, J. L., & Kupper, L. L. (2003). Substance use before and during pregnancy: Links to intimate partner violence. *The American Journal of Drug and Alcohol Abuse, 29,* 599–617. http://dx.doi.org/10.1081/ADA-120023461

Martins, S. S., Sarvet, A., Santaella-Tenorio, J., Saha, T., Grant, B. F., & Hasin, D. S. (2017). Changes in US lifetime heroin use and heroin use disorder: Prevalence from the 2001–2002 to 2012–2013 National Epidemiologic Survey on Alcohol and Related Conditions. *JAMA Psychiatry, 74,* 445–455. http://dx.doi.org/10.1001/jamapsychiatry.2017.0113

Mastin, D. F., Bryson, J., & Corwyn, R. (2006). Assessment of sleep hygiene using the Sleep Hygiene Index. *Journal of Behavioral Medicine, 29,* 223–227. http://dx.doi.org/10.1007/s10865-006-9047-6

McCabe, S. E., Hughes, T. L., Bostwick, W. B., West, B. T., & Boyd, C. J. (2009). Sexual orientation, substance use behaviors and substance dependence in the United States. *Addiction, 104,* 1333–1345. http://dx.doi.org/10.1111/j.1360-0443.2009.02596.x

McCabe, S. E., & West, B. T. (2013). Medical and nonmedical use of prescription stimulants: Results from a national multicohort study. *Journal of the American Academy of Child & Adolescent Psychiatry, 52,* 1272–1280. http://dx.doi.org/10.1016/j.jaac.2013.09.005

McCabe, S. E., & West, B. T. (2014). Medical and nonmedical use of prescription benzodiazepine anxiolytics among U.S. high school seniors. *Addictive Behaviors, 39,* 959–964. http://dx.doi.org/10.1016/j.addbeh.2014.01.009

McCabe, S. E., West, B. T., Teter, C. J., & Boyd, C. J. (2012). Medical and nonmedical use of prescription opioids among high school seniors in the United States. *Archives of Pediatrics & Adolescent Medicine, 166,* 797–802. http://dx.doi.org/10.1001/archpediatrics.2012.85

McCarthy, E., & Petrakis, I. (2011). Case report on the use of cognitive processing therapy-cognitive, enhanced to address heavy alcohol use. *Journal of Traumatic Stress, 24,* 474–478. http://dx.doi.org/10.1002/jts.20660

McCrady, B. S., & Epstein, E. E. (2009). *Overcoming alcohol problems: A couples-focused program.* New York, NY: Oxford University Press.

McKay, J. R. (2009). *Treating substance use disorders with adaptive continuing care.* Washington, DC: American Psychological Association. http://dx.doi.org/10.1037/11888-000

McKay, J. R., Alterman, A. I., Cacciola, J. S., O'Brien, C. P., Koppenhaver, J. M., & Shepard, D. S. (1999). Continuing care for cocaine dependence: Comprehensive 2-year outcomes. *Journal of Consulting and Clinical Psychology, 67,* 420–427. http://dx.doi.org/10.1037/0022-006X.67.3.420

McKay, J. R., Van Horn, D. H., Oslin, D. W., Lynch, K. G., Ivey, M., Ward, K., . . . Coviello, D. M. (2010). A randomized trial of extended telephone-based continuing care for alcohol dependence: Within-treatment substance use outcomes. *Journal of Consulting and Clinical Psychology, 78,* 912–923. http://dx.doi.org/10.1037/a0020700

McLarnon, M. E., Monaghan, T. L., Stewart, S. H., & Barrett, S. P. (2011). Drug misuse and diversion in adults prescribed anxiolytics and sedatives. *Pharmacotherapy, 31,* 262–272. http://dx.doi.org/10.1592/phco.31.3.262

McLean, C. P., Asnaani, A., Litz, B. T., & Hofmann, S. G. (2011). Gender differences in anxiety disorders: Prevalence, course of illness, comorbidity and burden of illness. *Journal of Psychiatric Research, 45*, 1027–1035. http://dx.doi.org/10.1016/j.jpsychires.2011.03.006

McLellan, A. T., Lewis, D. C., O'Brien, C. P., & Kleber, H. D. (2000). Drug dependence, a chronic medical illness: Implications for treatment, insurance, and outcomes evaluation. *JAMA, 284*, 1689–1695. http://dx.doi.org/10.1001/jama.284.13.1689

Mee-Lee, D., Shulman, G. D., Fishman, M. J., Gastfriend, D. R., & Miller, M. M. (Eds.). (2013). *The ASAM criteria: Treatment criteria for addictive, substance-related, and co-occurring conditions* (3rd ed.). Carson City, NV: The Change Companies.

Meyers, R. J., Miller, W. R., Hill, D. E., & Tonigan, J. S. (1998). Community reinforcement and family training (CRAFT): Engaging unmotivated drug users in treatment. *Journal of Substance Abuse, 10*, 291–308. http://dx.doi.org/10.1016/S0899-3289(99)00003-6

Meyers, R. J., & Wolfe, B. L. (2003). *Get your loved one sober: Alternatives to nagging, pleading, and threatening.* Center City, MN: Hazelden.

Miller, W. R., & Brown, S. A. (1997). Why psychologists should treat alcohol and drug problems. *American Psychologist, 52*, 1269–1279. http://dx.doi.org/10.1037/0003-066X.52.12.1269

Miller, W. R., Meyers, R. J., & Tonigan, J. S. (1999). Engaging the unmotivated in treatment for alcohol problems: A comparison of three strategies for intervention through family members. *Journal of Consulting and Clinical Psychology, 67*, 688–697. http://dx.doi.org/10.1037/0022-006X.67.5.688

Miller, W. R., & Rollnick, S. (2013). *Motivational interviewing: Helping people change* (3rd ed.). New York, NY: Guilford Press.

Miller, W. R., Zweben, A., DiClemente, C. C., & Rychtarik, R. G. (1999). Motivational enhancement therapy manual: A clinical research guide for therapists treating individuals with alcohol abuse and dependence. In M. E. Mattson (Series Ed.), *Project MATCH Monograph Series* (Vol. 2, NIH Publication No. 94-3723). Rockville, MD: National Institute on Alcohol Abuse and Alcoholism. Retrieved from https://pubs.niaaa.nih.gov/publications/ProjectMatch/match02.pdf

Mills, K. L., Teesson, M., Back, S. E., Brady, K. T., Baker, A. L., Hopwood, S., . . . Ewer, P. L. (2012). Integrated exposure-based therapy for co-occurring posttraumatic stress disorder and substance dependence: A randomized controlled trial. *JAMA, 308*, 690–699. http://dx.doi.org/10.1001/jama.2012.9071

Moos, R. H., & Moos, B. S. (2007). Treated and untreated alcohol-use disorders: Course and predictors of remission and relapse. *Evaluation Review, 31*, 564–584. http://dx.doi.org/10.1177/0193841X07306749

Morgenthaler, T., Kramer, M., Alessi, C., Friedman, L., Boehlecke, B., Brown, T., . . . Swick, T., & the American Academy of Sleep Medicine. (2006).

Practice parameters for the psychological and behavioral treatment of insomnia: An update. An American Academy of Sleep Medicine report. *Sleep, 29,* 1415–1419. http://dx.doi.org/10.1093/sleep/29.11.1415

Morin, C. M. (1993). *Insomnia: Psychological assessment and management.* New York, NY: Guilford Press.

Morin, C. M., & Espie, C. A. (2004). *Insomnia: A clinical guide to assessment and treatment.* New York, NY: Springer Science + Business Media.

Morin, C. M., Hauri, P. J., Espie, C. A., Spielman, A. J., Buysse, D. J., & Bootzin, R. R. (1999). Nonpharmacologic treatment of chronic insomnia. An American Academy of Sleep Medicine review. *Sleep, 22,* 1134–1156. http://dx.doi.org/10.1093/sleep/22.8.1134

Moyer, V. A., & U.S. Preventive Services Task Force. (2013). Screening and behavioral counseling interventions in primary care to reduce alcohol misuse: U.S. Preventive Services Task Force recommendation statement. *Annals of Internal Medicine, 159,* 210–218. http://dx.doi.org/10.7326/0003-4819-159-3-201308060-00652

National Academies of Sciences, Engineering, and Medicine. (2017). *The health effects of cannabis and cannabinoids: The current state of evidence and recommendations for research.* Washington, DC: The National Academies Press. http://dx.doi.org/10.17226/24625

National Institute on Alcohol Abuse and Alcoholism. (2003). *Assessing alcohol problems: A guide for clinicians and researchers* (2nd ed., NIH Publication No. 03-3745). Retrieved from https://pubs.niaaa.nih.gov/publications/guide.htm

National Institute on Alcohol Abuse and Alcoholism. (2010). *Rethinking drinking: Alcohol and your health* (NIH Publication No. 10-3770). Retrieved from https://pubs.niaaa.nih.gov/publications/rethinkingdrinking/rethinking_drinking.pdf

National Institute on Drug Abuse. (2012a). *Research Report Series: Inhalants* (NIH Publication No. 12-3818). Retrieved from https://www.drugabuse.gov/publications/research-reports/inhalants

National Institute on Drug Abuse. (2012b). *Resource guide: Screening for drug use in general medical settings.* Retrieved from https://www.drugabuse.gov/publications/resource-guide-screening-drug-use-in-general-medical-settings/

National Institute on Drug Abuse. (2013). *Research Report Series: Methamphetamine* (NIH Publication No. 13-4210). Retrieved from https://www.drugabuse.gov/publications/research-reports/methamphetamine

National Institute on Drug Abuse. (2014). *Drugs, brains, and behavior: The science of addiction.* Retrieved from https://www.drugabuse.gov/sites/default/files/soa_2014.pdf

National Institute on Drug Abuse. (2015). *Research Report Series: Hallucinogens and dissociative drugs* (NIH Publication No. 15-4209). Retrieved from https://www.drugabuse.gov/publications/research-reports/hallucinogens-dissociative-drugs

National Institute on Drug Abuse. (2016). *Research Report Series: Cocaine.* Retrieved from https://www.drugabuse.gov/publications/research-reports/cocaine

National Institute on Drug Abuse. (2017). *Research Report Series: MDMA (ecstasy) abuse.* Retrieved from https://www.drugabuse.gov/publications/research-reports/mdma-ecstasy-abuse

National Institute on Drug Abuse. (2018a). *Prescription stimulants.* Retrieved from https://www.drugabuse.gov/publications/drugfacts/prescription-stimulants

National Institute on Drug Abuse. (2018b). *Principles of drug addiction treatment: A research-based guide* (3rd ed.). Bethesda, MD: National Institute on Drug Abuse; National Institutes of Health; U.S. Department of Health and Human Services.

National Institute on Drug Abuse. (2018c). *Research Report Series: Misuse of prescription drugs.* Retrieved from https://www.drugabuse.gov/publications/research-reports/misuse-prescription-drugs

National Public Radio. (2007). *Prozac the most widely used antidepressant.* Retrieved from https://www.npr.org/templates/story/story.php?storyId=10253841

National Sleep Foundation. (2019). *The sleep disorders.* Retrieved from http://sleepdisorders.sleepfoundation.org/

Nestler, E. J. (2005). Is there a common molecular pathway for addiction? *Nature Neuroscience, 8,* 1445–1449. http://dx.doi.org/10.1038/nn1578

Neutel, C. I. (2005). The epidemiology of long-term benzodiazepine use. *International Review of Psychiatry, 17,* 189–197. http://dx.doi.org/10.1080/09540260500071863

Norton, G. R., Norton, P. J., Cox, B. J., & Belik, S.-L. (2008). Panic spectrum disorders and substance use. In S. H. Stewart & P. J. Conrod (Eds.), A*nxiety and substance abuse disorders: The vicious cycle of comorbidity* (pp. 81–98). New York, NY: Springer. http://dx.doi.org/10.1007/978-0-387-74290-8_5

Nowinski, J., Baker, S., & Carroll, K. (1999). Twelve step facilitation therapy manual: A clinical research guide for therapists treating individuals with alcohol abuse and dependence. In M. E. Mattson (Series Ed.), *Project MATCH Monograph Series* (Vol. 1, NIH Publication No. 94-3722). Rockville, MD: National Institute on Alcohol Abuse and Alcoholism. Retrieved from https://pubs.niaaa.nih.gov/publications/projectmatch/match01.pdf

Nunes, E. V., & Levin, F. R. (2004). Treatment of depression in patients with alcohol or other drug dependence: A meta-analysis. *JAMA, 291,* 1887–1896. http://dx.doi.org/10.1001/jama.291.15.1887

O'Farrell, T. J., & Clements, K. (2012). Review of outcome research on marital and family therapy in treatment for alcoholism. *Journal of Marital and Family Therapy, 38,* 122–144. http://dx.doi.org/10.1111/j.1752-0606.2011.00242.x

O'Farrell, T. J., & Fals-Stewart, W. (2003). Alcohol abuse. *Journal of Marital and Family Therapy, 29,* 121–146. http://dx.doi.org/10.1111/j.1752-0606.2003.tb00387.x

Olatunji, B. O., Cisler, J. M., & Deacon, B. J. (2010). Efficacy of cognitive behavioral therapy for anxiety disorders: A review of meta-analytic findings. *Psychiatric Clinics of North America, 33*, 557–577. http://dx.doi.org/10.1016/j.psc.2010.04.002

Ondersma, S. J., Simpson, S. M., Brestan, E. V., & Ward, M. (2000). Prenatal drug exposure and social policy: The search for an appropriate response. *Child Maltreatment, 5*, 93–108. http://dx.doi.org/10.1177/1077559500005002002

Orford, J., Velleman, R., Natera, G., Templeton, L., & Copello, A. (2013). Addiction in the family is a major but neglected contributor to the global burden of adult ill-health. *Social Science & Medicine, 78*, 70–77. http://dx.doi.org/10.1016/j.socscimed.2012.11.036

Osborn, L. A., Lauritsen, K. J., Cross, N., Davis, A. K., Rosenberg, H., Bonadio, F., & Lang, B. (2015). Self-medication of somatic and psychiatric conditions using botanical marijuana. *Journal of Psychoactive Drugs, 47*, 345–350. http://dx.doi.org/10.1080/02791072.2015.1096433

Ougrin, D. (2011). Efficacy of exposure versus cognitive therapy in anxiety disorders: Systematic review and meta-analysis. *BMC Psychiatry, 11*, 200. http://dx.doi.org/10.1186/1471-244X-11-200

Pagnini, D. L., & Reichman, N. E. (2000). Psychosocial factors and the timing of prenatal care among women in New Jersey's HealthStart program. *Family Planning Perspectives, 32*(2), 56–64. http://dx.doi.org/10.2307/2648213

Pasala, S., Barr, T., & Messaoudi, I. (2015). Impact of alcohol abuse on the adaptive immune system. *Alcohol Research: Current Reviews, 37*, 185–197.

Perlis, M. L., Jungquist, C., Smith, M. T., & Posner, D. (2005). *Cognitive behavioral treatment of insomnia: A session-by-session guide.* New York, NY: Springer.

Peters, E. N., Khondkaryan, E., & Sullivan, T. P. (2012). Associations between expectancies of alcohol and drug use, severity of partner violence, and posttraumatic stress among women. *Journal of Interpersonal Violence, 27*, 2108–2127. http://dx.doi.org/10.1177/0886260511432151

Petry, N. M. (2000). A comprehensive guide to the application of contingency management procedures in clinical settings. *Drug and Alcohol Dependence, 58*, 9–25. http://dx.doi.org/10.1016/S0376-8716(99)00071-X

Pettinati, H. M. (2004). Antidepressant treatment of co-occurring depression and alcohol dependence. *Biological Psychiatry, 56*, 785–792. http://dx.doi.org/10.1016/j.biopsych.2004.07.016

Pettinati, H. M., O'Brien, C. P., & Dundon, W. D. (2013). Current status of co-occurring mood and substance use disorders: A new therapeutic target. *The American Journal of Psychiatry, 170*, 23–30. http://dx.doi.org/10.1176/appi.ajp.2012.12010112

Platt, L., Melendez-Torres, G. J., O'Donnell, A., Bradley, J., Newbury-Birch, D., Kaner, E., & Ashton, C. (2016). How effective are brief interventions in reducing alcohol consumption: Do the setting, practitioner group and content matter? Findings from a systematic review and metaregression analysis. *BMJ Open, 6*, e011473. http://dx.doi.org/10.1136/bmjopen-2016-011473

Pringle, J. L., Kowalchuk, A., Meyers, J. A., & Seale, J. P. (2012). Equipping residents to address alcohol and drug abuse: The national SBIRT residency training project. *Journal of Graduate Medical Education, 4*, 58–63. http://dx.doi.org/10.4300/JGME-D-11-00019.1

Prochaska, J. O., DiClemente, C. C., & Norcross, J. C. (1992). In search of how people change. Applications to addictive behaviors. *American Psychologist, 47*, 1102–1114. http://dx.doi.org/10.1037/0003-066X.47.9.1102

Project Match Research Group. (1997). Matching alcoholism treatments to client heterogeneity: Project MATCH posttreatment drinking outcomes. *Journal of Studies on Alcohol, 58*, 7–29. http://dx.doi.org/10.15288/jsa.1997.58.7

Project Match Research Group. (1998). Matching alcoholism treatments to client heterogeneity: Project MATCH three-year drinking outcomes. *Alcoholism: Clinician and Experimental Research, 22*, 1300–1311.

Radloff, L. S. (1977). The CES-D scale: A self-report depression scale for research in the general population. *Applied Psychological Measurement, 1*, 385–401. http://dx.doi.org/10.1177/014662167700100306

Rahm, A. K., Boggs, J. M., Martin, C., Price, D. W., Beck, A., Backer, T. E., & Dearing, J. W. (2015). Facilitators and barriers to implementing Screening, Brief Intervention, and Referral to Treatment (SBIRT) in primary care in integrated health care settings. *Substance Abuse, 36*, 281–288. http://dx.doi.org/10.1080/08897077.2014.951140

Ram, S., Seirawan, H., Kumar, S. K. S., & Clark, G. T. (2010). Prevalence and impact of sleep disorders and sleep habits in the United States. *Sleep and Breathing, 14*, 63–70. http://dx.doi.org/10.1007/s11325-009-0281-3

Randall, C. L., Thomas, S., & Thevos, A. K. (2001). Concurrent alcoholism and social anxiety disorder: A first step toward developing effective treatments. *Alcoholism: Clinical and Experimental Research, 25*, 210–220. http://dx.doi.org/10.1111/j.1530-0277.2001.tb02201.x

Read, J. P., Bollinger, A. R., & Sharkansky, E. (2003). Assessment of comorbid substance use disorder and posttraumatic stress disorder. In P. Ouimette & P. J. Brown (Eds.), *Trauma and substance abuse: Causes, consequences, and treatment of comorbid disorders* (pp. 111–125). Washington, DC: American Psychological Association. http://dx.doi.org/10.1037/10460-006

Rehm, J., Mathers, C., Popova, S., Thavorncharoensap, M., Teerawattananon, Y., & Patra, J. (2009). Global burden of disease and injury and economic cost attributable to alcohol use and alcohol-use disorders. *The Lancet, 373*, 2223–2233. http://dx.doi.org/10.1016/S0140-6736(09)60746-7

Reisfield, G. M., Webb, F. J., Bertholf, R. L., Sloan, P. A., & Wilson, G. R. (2007). Family physicians' proficiency in urine drug test interpretation. *Journal of Opioid Management, 3*, 333–337. http://dx.doi.org/10.5055/jom.2007.0022

Resick, P. A., Galovski, T. E., Uhlmansiek, M. O., Scher, C. D., Clum, G. A., & Young-Xu, Y. (2008). A randomized clinical trial to dismantle components of cognitive processing therapy for posttraumatic stress disorder in female victims of interpersonal violence. *Journal of Consulting and Clinical Psychology, 76*, 243–258. http://dx.doi.org/10.1037/0022-006X.76.2.243

Resick, P. A., Nishith, P., Weaver, T. L., Astin, M. C., & Feuer, C. A. (2002). A comparison of cognitive-processing therapy with prolonged exposure and a waiting condition for the treatment of chronic posttraumatic stress disorder in female rape victims. *Journal of Consulting and Clinical Psychology, 70*, 867–879. http://dx.doi.org/10.1037/0022-006X.70.4.867

Richter, L., Pugh, B. S., Peters, E. A., Vaughan, R. D., & Foster, S. E. (2016). Underage drinking: Prevalence and correlates of risky drinking measures among youth aged 12–20. *The American Journal of Drug and Alcohol Abuse, 42*, 385–394. http://dx.doi.org/10.3109/00952990.2015.1102923

Riper, H., Andersson, G., Hunter, S. B., de Wit, J., Berking, M., & Cuijpers, P. (2014). Treatment of comorbid alcohol use disorders and depression with cognitive-behavioural therapy and motivational interviewing: A meta-analysis. *Addiction, 109*, 394–406. http://dx.doi.org/10.1111/add.12441

Roane, B. M., & Taylor, D. J. (2008). Adolescent insomnia as a risk factor for early adult depression and substance abuse. *Sleep, 31*, 1351–1356.

Roberts, N. P., Roberts, P. A., Jones, N., & Bisson, J. I. (2016). Psychological therapies for post-traumatic stress disorder and comorbid substance use disorder. *Cochrane Database of Systematic Reviews, 4*, CD010204. Advance online publication. http://dx.doi.org/10.1002/14651858.CD010204.pub2

Robinson, J., Sareen, J., Cox, B. J., & Bolton, J. M. (2011). Role of self-medication in the development of comorbid anxiety and substance use disorders: A longitudinal investigation. *Archives of General Psychiatry, 68*, 800–807. http://dx.doi.org/10.1001/archgenpsychiatry.2011.75

Rockett, I. R. H., Putnam, S. L., Jia, H., & Smith, G. S. (2006). Declared and undeclared substance use among emergency department patients: A population-based study. *Addiction, 101*, 706–712. http://dx.doi.org/10.1111/j.1360-0443.2006.01397.x

Roehrs, T. A., & Roth, T. (2001). Sleep, sleepiness, and alcohol use. *Alcohol Research and Health, 25*, 101–109.

Roehrs, T. A., & Roth, T. (2015). Sleep disturbance in substance use disorders. *Psychiatric Clinics of North America, 38*, 793–803. http://dx.doi.org/10.1016/j.psc.2015.07.008

Roerecke, M., Tobe, S. W., Kaczorowski, J., Bacon, S. L., Vafaei, A., Hasan, O. S. M., . . . Rehm, J. (2018). Sex-specific associations between alcohol consumption and incidence of hypertension: A systematic review and meta-analysis of cohort studies. *Journal of the American Heart Association, 7*, 1–27. http://dx.doi.org/10.1161/JAHA.117.008202

Rohde, P., Lewinsohn, P. M., Kahler, C. W., Seeley, J. R., & Brown, R. A. (2001). Natural course of alcohol use disorders from adolescence to young adulthood. *Journal of the American Academy of Child & Adolescent Psychiatry, 40*, 83–90. http://dx.doi.org/10.1097/00004583-200101000-00020

Rollnick, S., Miller, W. R., & Butler, C. C. (2007). *Motivational interviewing in health care: Helping patients change behavior.* New York, NY: Guilford Press.

Roozen, H. G., de Waart, R., & van der Kroft, P. (2010). Community reinforcement and family training: An effective option to engage treatment-resistant substance-abusing individuals in treatment. *Addiction, 105,* 1729–1738. http://dx.doi.org/10.1111/j.1360-0443.2010.03016.x

Rosen, C. S., Henson, B. R., Finney, J. W., & Moos, R. H. (2000). Consistency of self-administered and interview-based Addiction Severity Index composite scores. *Addiction, 95,* 419–425. http://dx.doi.org/10.1046/j.1360-0443.2000.95341912.x

Rubinsky, A. D., Kivlahan, D. R., Volk, R. J., Maynard, C., & Bradley, K. A. (2010). Estimating risk of alcohol dependence using alcohol screening scores. *Drug and Alcohol Dependence, 108,* 29–36. http://dx.doi.org/10.1016/j.drugalcdep.2009.11.009

Saha, T. D., Kerridge, B. T., Goldstein, R. B., Chou, S. P., Zhang, H., Jung, J., . . . Grant, B. F. (2016). Nonmedical prescription opioid use and *DSM–5* nonmedical prescription opioid use disorder in the United States. *The Journal of Clinical Psychiatry, 77,* 772–780. http://dx.doi.org/10.4088/JCP.15m10386

Saitz, R. (2013). Confidentiality. In R. Saitz (Ed.), *Addressing alcohol use in primary care.* New York, NY: Springer. http://dx.doi.org/10.1007/978-1-4614-4779-5_16

Saitz, R., Palfai, T. P., Cheng, D. M., Alford, D. P., Bernstein, J. A., Lloyd-Travaglini, C. A., . . . Samet, J. H. (2014). Screening and brief intervention for drug use in primary care: The ASPIRE randomized controlled trial. *JAMA, 312,* 502–513. http://dx.doi.org/10.1001/jama.2014.7862

Schaeffer, T. (2012). Abuse-deterrent formulations, an evolving technology against the abuse and misuse of opioid analgesics. *Journal of Medical Toxicology, 8,* 400–407. http://dx.doi.org/10.1007/s13181-012-0270-y

Schepis, T. S., & McCabe, S. E. (2016). Trends in older adult nonmedical prescription drug use prevalence: Results from the 2002–2003 and 2012–2013 National Survey on Drug Use and Health. *Addictive Behaviors, 60,* 219–222. http://dx.doi.org/10.1016/j.addbeh.2016.04.020

Schumacher, J. A., Feldbau-Kohn, S., Slep, A. M. S., & Heyman, R. E. (2001). Risk factors for male-to-female partner physical abuse. *Aggression and Violent Behavior, 6,* 281–352. http://dx.doi.org/10.1016/S1359-1789(00)00027-6

Schumacher, J. A., & Holt, D. J. (2012). Domestic violence shelter residents' substance abuse treatment needs and options. *Aggression and Violent Behavior, 17,* 188–197. http://dx.doi.org/10.1016/j.avb.2012.01.002

Schumacher, J. A., & Madson, M. B. (2015). *Fundamental of motivational interviewing: Tips and strategies for addressing common clinical challenges.* New York, NY: Oxford University Press.

Schumacher, J. A., Stafford, P. A., Beadnell, B., & Crisafulli, M. (2018). A comparison by age of adults in indicated prevention following impaired driving.

Journal of Addictions & Offender Counseling, 39, 106–126. http://dx.doi.org/10.1002/jaoc.12050

Serafini, G., Howland, R. H., Rovedi, F., Girardi, P., & Amore, M. (2014). The role of ketamine in treatment-resistant depression: A systematic review. *Current Neuropharmacology, 12,* 444–461. http://dx.doi.org/10.2174/1570159X12666140619204251

Sessa, B. (2011). Could MDMA be useful in the treatment of post-traumatic stress disorder? *Progress in Neurology and Psychiatry, 15,* 4–7. http://dx.doi.org/10.1002/pnp.216

Singla, S., Sachdeva, R., & Mehta, J. L. (2012). Cannabinoids and athero-sclerotic coronary heart disease. *Clinical Cardiology, 35,* 329–335. http://dx.doi.org/10.1002/clc.21962

Skinner, H. A. (1982). The drug abuse screening test. *Addictive Behaviors, 7,* 363–371. http://dx.doi.org/10.1016/0306-4603(82)90005-3

Skinner, M. D., Lahmek, P., Pham, H., & Aubin, H. J. (2014). Disulfiram efficacy in the treatment of alcohol dependence: A meta-analysis. *PLoS One, 9,* e87366. http://dx.doi.org/10.1371/journal.pone.0087366

Smith, J. P., & Randall, C. L. (2012). Anxiety and alcohol use disorders: Comorbidity and treatment considerations. *Alcohol Research: Current Reviews, 34,* 414–431.

Smith, P. C., Schmidt, S. M., Allensworth-Davies, D., & Saitz, R. (2009). Primary care validation of a single-question alcohol screening test. *Journal of General Internal Medicine, 24,* 783–788. http://dx.doi.org/10.1007/s11606-009-0928-6

Smith, P. C., Schmidt, S. M., Allensworth-Davies, D., & Saitz, R. (2010). A single-question screening test for drug use in primary care. *Archives of Internal Medicine, 170,* 1155–1160. http://dx.doi.org/10.1001/archinternmed.2010.140

Spielman, A. J., Caruso, L. S., & Glovinsky, P. B. (1987). A behavioral perspective on insomnia treatment. *Psychiatric Clinics of North America, 10,* 541–553. http://dx.doi.org/10.1016/S0193-953X(18)30532-X

Spitzer, R. L., Kroenke, K., Williams, J. B., & Löwe, B. (2006). A brief measure for assessing generalized anxiety disorder: The GAD-7. *Archives of Internal Medicine, 166,* 1092–1097. http://dx.doi.org/10.1001/archinte.166.10.1092

Stewart, S. H., & Conrod, P. J. (2008). Anxiety disorder and substance use disorder co-morbidity: Common themes and future directions. In S. H. Stewart & P. J. Conrod (Eds.), *Anxiety and substance abuse disorders: The vicious cycle of comorbidity* (pp. 239–257). New York, NY: Springer. http://dx.doi.org/10.1007/978-0-387-74290-8_13

Substance Abuse and Mental Health Services Administration. (2013). *Results from the 2012 National Survey on Drug Use and Health: Summary of national findings.* Retrieved from https://www.samhsa.gov/data/sites/default/files/NSDUHresults2012/NSDUHresults2012.pdf

Substance Abuse and Mental Health Services Administration. (2014). Treating sleep problems of people in recovery from substance use disorders. *In Brief, 8*(2). Retrieved from https://store.samhsa.gov/system/files/sma14-4859.pdf

Substance Abuse and Mental Health Services Administration. (2017). *Key substance use and mental health indicators in the United States: Results from the 2016 National Survey on Drug Use and Health* (HHS Publication No. SMA 17-5044, NSDUH Series H-52). Retrieved from https://www.samhsa.gov/data/sites/default/files/NSDUH-FFR1-2016/NSDUH-FFR1-2016.htm

Swendsen, J., Conway, K. P., Degenhardt, L., Glantz, M., Jin, R., Merikangas, K. R., . . . Kessler, R. C. (2010). Mental disorders as risk factors for substance use, abuse and dependence: Results from the 10-year follow-up of the National Comorbidity Survey. *Addiction, 105,* 1117–1128. http://dx.doi.org/10.1111/j.1360-0443.2010.02902.x

Tan, P. D., Barclay, J. S., & Blackhall, L. J. (2015). Do palliative care clinics screen for substance abuse and diversion? Results of a national survey. *Journal of Palliative Medicine, 18,* 752–757. http://dx.doi.org/10.1089/jpm.2015.0098

Teter, C. J., McCabe, S. E., LaGrange, K., Cranford, J. A., & Boyd, C. J. (2006). Illicit use of specific prescription stimulants among college students: Prevalence, motives, and routes of administration. *Pharmacotherapy, 26,* 1501–1510. http://dx.doi.org/10.1592/phco.26.10.1501

Thomas, G., Kloner, R. A., & Rezkalla, S. (2014). Adverse cardiovascular, cerebrovascular, and peripheral vascular effects of marijuana inhalation: What cardiologists need to know. *The American Journal of Cardiology, 113,* 187–190. http://dx.doi.org/10.1016/j.amjcard.2013.09.042

Timko, C., Laudet, A., & Moos, R. H. (2016). Al-Anon newcomers: Benefits of continuing attendance for six months. *The American Journal of Drug and Alcohol Abuse, 42,* 441–449. http://dx.doi.org/10.3109/00952990.2016.1148702

Timko, C., Young, L. B., & Moos, R. H. (2012). Al-Anon family groups: Origins, conceptual basis, outcomes, and research opportunities. *Journal of Groups in Addiction & Recovery, 7,* 279–296. http://dx.doi.org/10.1080/1556035X.2012.705713

Toma, A., Paré, G., & Leong, D. P. (2017). Alcohol and cardiovascular disease: How much is too much? *Current Atherosclerosis Reports, 19,* 13. http://dx.doi.org/10.1007/s11883-017-0647-0

Toneatto, T., & Rector, N. A. (2008). Treating co-morbid panic disorder and substance use disorder. In S. H. Stewart & P. J. Conrod (Eds.), *Anxiety and substance abuse disorders: The vicious cycle of comorbidity* (pp. 157–175). New York, NY: Springer. http://dx.doi.org/10.1007/978-0-387-74290-8_9

Tonigan, J. S., Pearson, M. R., Magill, M., & Hagler, K. J. (2018). AA attendance and abstinence for dually diagnosed patients: A meta-analytic review. *Addiction, 113,* 1970–1981. http://dx.doi.org/10.1111/add.14268

Trauer, J. M., Qian, M. Y., Doyle, J. S. W., Rajaratnam, S. M., & Cunnington, D. (2015). Cognitive behavioral therapy for chronic insomnia: A systematic review and meta-analysis. *Annals of Internal Medicine, 163,* 191–204. http://dx.doi.org/10.7326/M14-2841

U.S. Department of Health and Human Services, & U.S. Department of Agriculture. (2015). *Dietary Guidelines 2015–2020: Appendix 9. Alcohol.* Retrieved from https://health.gov/dietaryguidelines/2015/guidelines/appendix-9/

U.S. Preventive Services Task Force. (2019, May). *Final recommendation statement: Tobacco smoking cessation in adults, including pregnant women: Behavioral and pharmacotherapy interventions.* Retrieved from https://www.uspreventiveservicestaskforce.org/Page/Document/RecommendationStatementFinal/tobacco-use-in-adults-and-pregnant-women-counseling-and-interventions1

van der Pol, P., Liebregts, N., de Graaf, R., Korf, D. J., van den Brink, W., & van Laar, M. (2013). Predicting the transition from frequent cannabis use to cannabis dependence: A three-year prospective study. *Drug and Alcohol Dependence, 133,* 352–359. http://dx.doi.org/10.1016/j.drugalcdep.2013.06.009

Vendetti, J., Gmyrek, A., Damon, D., Singh, M., McRee, B., & Del Boca, F. (2017). Screening, brief intervention and referral to treatment (SBIRT): Implementation barriers, facilitators and model migration. *Addiction, 112*(Suppl. 2), 23–33. http://dx.doi.org/10.1111/add.13652

Veterans Affairs/Department of Defense. (2015). *Clinical practice guideline for the management of substance use disorders.* Retrieved from https://www.healthquality.va.gov/guidelines/MH/sud/VADoDSUDCPGRevised22216.pdf

Viel, G., Boscolo-Berto, R., Cecchetto, G., Fais, P., Nalesso, A., & Ferrara, S. D. (2012). Phosphatidylethanol in blood as a marker of chronic alcohol use: A systematic review and meta-analysis. *International Journal of Molecular Sciences, 13,* 14788–14812. http://dx.doi.org/10.3390/ijms131114788

Volkow, N. D., Baler, R. D., Compton, W. M., & Weiss, S. R. (2014). Adverse health effects of marijuana use. *The New England Journal of Medicine, 370,* 2219–2227. http://dx.doi.org/10.1056/NEJMra1402309

Volpicelli, J. R., Watson, N. T., King, A. C., Sherman, C. E., & O'Brien, C. P. (1995). Effect of naltrexone on alcohol "high" in alcoholics. *The American Journal of Psychiatry, 152,* 613–615. http://dx.doi.org/10.1176/ajp.152.4.613

Wasserman, D. A., Stewart, A. L., & Delucchi, K. L. (2001). Social support and abstinence from opiates and cocaine during opioid maintenance treatment. *Drug and Alcohol Dependence, 65,* 65–75. http://dx.doi.org/10.1016/S0376-8716(01)00151-X

Weathermon, R., & Crabb, D. W. (1999). Alcohol and medication interactions. *Alcohol Research & Health, 23,* 40–54.

Weaver, M. (2013). Choices for patients and clinicians: Ethics and legal issues. In R. Saitz (Ed.), *Addressing alcohol use in primary care.* New York, NY: Springer. http://dx.doi.org/10.1007/978-1-4614-4779-5_17

Weiss, R. D., Najavits, L. M., Greenfield, S. F., Soto, J. A., Shaw, S. R., & Wyner, D. (1998). Validity of substance use self-reports in dually diagnosed outpatients. *The American Journal of Psychiatry, 155,* 127–128. http://dx.doi.org/10.1176/ajp.155.1.127

Wickwire, E. M., Schumacher, J. A., & Clarke, E. J. (2009). Patient-reported benefits from the pre-sleep routine approach to treating insomnia. Findings from a treatment development trial. *Sleep and Biological Rhythms, 7*(2), 71–77. http://dx.doi.org/10.1111/j.1479-8425.2009.00389.x

Wilson, J. M. G., & Jungner, G. (1968). *Principles and practices of screening for disease.* Geneva, Switzerland: World Health Organization. Retrieved from http://www.who.int/ionizing_radiation/medical_radiation_exposure/munich-WHO-1968-Screening-Disease.pdf

Wong, M. M., Brower, K. J., Nigg, J. T., & Zucker, R. A. (2010). Childhood sleep problems, response inhibition, and alcohol and drug outcomes in adolescence and young adulthood. *Alcoholism: Clinical and Experimental Research, 34,* 1033–1044. http://dx.doi.org/10.1111/j.1530-0277.2010.01178.x

Wood, E., Albarquoni, L., Tkachuk, S., Green, C. J., Ahmad, K., Nolan, S., . . . Klimas, J. (2018). Will this hospitalized patient develop severe alcohol withdrawal syndrome? The rational clinical examination systematic review. *JAMA, 8,* 825–833. http://dx.doi.org/10.1001/jama.2018.10574

World Health Organization. (1992). *International classification of diseases and related health problems* (10th rev.). Geneva, Switzerland: Author.

World Health Organization. (2010). *The alcohol, smoking and substance involvement screening test (ASSIST): Manual for use in primary care.* Geneva, Switzerland: Author.

World Health Organization. (2014). *Global status report on alcohol and health—2014.* Geneva, Switzerland: World Health Organization. Retrieved from http://www.who.int/substance_abuse/publications/global_alcohol_report/en/

World Health Organization ASSIST Working Group. (2002). The Alcohol, Smoking and Substance Involvement Screening Test (ASSIST): Development, reliability and feasibility. *Addiction, 97,* 1183–1194. http://dx.doi.org/10.1046/j.1360-0443.2002.00185.x

Xu, Y., Hackett, M., Carter, G., Loo, C., Gálvez, V., Glozier, N., . . . Rodgers, A. (2016). Effects of low-dose and very low-dose Ketamine among patients with major depression: A systematic review and meta-analysis. *International Journal of Neuropsychopharmacology, 19,* pyv124. Advance online publication. http://dx.doi.org/10.1093/ijnp/pyv124

Zacny, J., Bigelow, G., Compton, P., Foley, K., Iguchi, M., & Sannerud, C. (2003). College on Problems of Drug Dependence taskforce on prescription opioid non-medical use and abuse: Position statement. *Drug and Alcohol Dependence, 69,* 215–232. http://dx.doi.org/10.1016/S0376-8716(03)00003-6

Zgierska, A., Rabago, D., Chawla, N., Kushner, K., Koehler, R., & Marlatt, A. (2009). Mindfulness meditation for substance use disorders: A systematic review. *Substance Abuse, 30,* 266–294. http://dx.doi.org/10.1080/08897070903250019

Zvolensky, M. J., Bernstein, A., Sachs-Ericsson, N., Schmidt, N. B., Buckner, J. D., & Bonn-Miller, M. O. (2006). Lifetime associations between cannabis, use, abuse, and dependence and panic attacks in a representative sample. *Journal of Psychiatric Research, 40,* 477–486. http://dx.doi.org/10.1016/j.jpsychires.2005.09.005

Index

About the Authors

Julie A. Schumacher, PhD, is a licensed clinical psychologist who completed her doctoral training at Stony Brook University and postdoctoral fellowship at the Research Institute on Addictions. For the past 15 years she has been on the faculty in the Department of Psychiatry and Human Behavior at the University of Mississippi Medical Center, where she currently serves as vice chair for education and also briefly held positions as research scientist at the Research Institute on Addictions and director of research at the Prevention Research Institute. Over the course of her career, she has (a) helped create and supervise a training experience for psychology interns and fellows located at a community-based substance use disorder treatment facility; (b) worked with her coauthor and other colleagues to implement curricula to provide training to psychology interns and fellows in motivational interviewing for substance use disorders and to provide training to medical students, psychiatry residents, nurses, and psychology interns in screening, brief intervention, and referral to treatment for alcohol and drugs; (c) treated or supervised treatment for numerous individuals struggling with their own or a loved one's harmful substance use; (d) maintained an active program of research primarily focused on the intersection of substance use, violence, and trauma, some of which is presented in this book; and most recently (e) become involved in various task forces, grant applications, and curriculum development efforts aimed at addressing the opioid crisis.

Daniel C. Williams, PhD, is a licensed clinical psychologist who completed his doctoral training at the University of Memphis and his internship at the Veterans Affairs (VA) North Texas Health Care System. Following internship he accepted a position as a psychologist in the Addictive Disorders Treatment Program at the VA Medical Center in Jackson, Mississippi, where he spent nearly a decade growing and developing evidence-based treatment programs for veterans; serving in mental health leadership positions; disseminating evidence-based addiction treatments to psychology trainees, psychologists, and other mental health providers; and providing consultation on mental health services in VA medical centers. More recently, he has continued this work as an associate professor, vice director of psychology training, and director of the Division of Psychology at the University of Mississippi Medical Center, where he continues, often with his coauthor, training mental health and medical providers in the assessment and treatment of addiction.